Self-Neglect:
Challenges
for Helping Professionals

Self-Neglect: Challenges for Helping Professionals has been co-published simultaneously as *Journal of Elder Abuse & Neglect,* Volume 11, Number 2 1999.

The *Journal of Elder Abuse & Neglect*™ Monographic "Separates"

Below is a list of "separates," which in serials librarianship means a special issue simultaneously published as a special journal issue or double-issue *and* as a "separate" hardbound monograph. (This is a format which we also call a "DocuSerial.")

"Separates" are published because specialized libraries or professionals may wish to purchase a specific thematic issue by itself in a format which can be separately cataloged and shelved, as opposed to purchasing the journal on an on-going basis. Faculty members may also more easily consider a "separate" for classroom adoption.

"Separates" are carefully classified separately with the major book jobbers so that the journal tie-in can be noted on new book order slips to avoid duplicate purchasing.

You may wish to visit Haworth's Website at . . .

http://www.haworthpressinc.com

. . . to search our online catalog for complete tables of contents of these separates and related publications.

You may also call 1-800-HAWORTH (outside US/Canada: 607-722-5857), or Fax 1-800-895-0582 (outside US/Canada: 607-771-0012), or e-mail at:

getinfo@haworthpressinc.com

Self-Neglect: **Challenges for Helping Professionals** edited by James G. O'Brien, MD (Vol. 11, No. 2, 1999).

Elder Abuse and Neglect in Residential Settings: Different National Backgrounds and Similar Responses, edited by Frank Glendenning, PhD, and Paul Kingston, PhD (Vol. 10, No. 1/2, 1999). *"This volume will help contribute to your greater understanding about the issues of elder abuse and neglect world-wide."*

Elder Mistreatment: Ethical Issues, Dilemmas, and Decisions, edited by Tanya Fusco Johnson, PhD, MDiv (Vol. 7, No. 2/3, 1995). *"I recommend this book to members of all health fields. It covers in depth the major ethical topics of autonomy, beneficence, legal competence, and justice, yet remains practical by discussing constraints to ideal solutions. Physical therapists who practice in home care and in nursing homes would find special benefit." (Physical Therapy)*

Elder Abuse: International and Cross-Cultural Perspectives, edited by Jordan I. Kosberg, PhD, and Juanita L. Garcia, EdD (Vol. 6, No. 3/4, 1995). *"A welcome and original contribution to the literature on elder abuse and is recommend reading for all with an interest in this field." (Age & Aging)*

Protecting Judgement-Impaired Adults: Issues, Interventions, and Policies, edited by Edmund F. Dejowski, JD, PhD (Vol. 2, No. 3/4, 1990). *"Provides eye-opening information about guardianship and alternative methods of serving judgement-impaired adults. . . . practical guidelines and suggestions for professional and nonprofessionals who find themselves involved with this population." (Adultspan)*

Self-Neglect: Challenges for Helping Professionals

James G. O'Brien, MD
Editor

Self-Neglect: Challenges for Helping Professionals has been co-published simultaneously as *Journal of Elder Abuse & Neglect*, Volume 11, Number 2 1999.

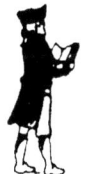

The Haworth Maltreatment & Trauma Press
An Imprint of
The Haworth Press, Inc.
New York • London • Oxford

Published by

The Haworth Maltreatment & Trauma Press, 10 Alice Street, Binghamton, NY 13904-1580 USA

The Haworth Maltreatment & Trauma Press is an Imprint of the Haworth Press, Inc., 10 Alice Street, Binghamton, NY 13904-1580 USA.

Self-Neglect: Challenges for Helping Professionals has also been published as *Journal of Elder Abuse & Neglect* Volume 11, Number 2 1999.

© 1999 by The Haworth Press, Inc. All rights reserved. No part of this work may be reproduced or utilized in any form or by any means, electronic or mechanical, including photocopying, microfilm and recording, or by any information storage and retrieval system, without permission in writing from the publisher. Printed in the United States of America.

The development, preparation, and publication of this work has been undertaken with great care. However, the publisher, employees, editors, and agents of The Haworth Press and all imprints of The Haworth Press, Inc., including The Haworth Medical Press and Pharmaceutical Products Press, are not responsible for any errors contained herein or for consequences that may ensue from use of materials or information contained in this work. Opinions expressed by the author(s) are not necessarily those of The Haworth Press, Inc.

The Haworth Press, Inc., 10 Alice Street, Binghamton, NY 13904-1580 USA

Cover design by Thomas J. Mayshock Jr.

Library of Congress Cataloging-in-Publication Data

Self-neglect : challenges for helping professionals / James G. O'Brien, editor.
    p. cm.
    Includes bibliographical references and index.
    ISBN 0-7890-0975-7 (alk. paper)–ISBN 0-7890-0993-5 (alk. paper)
    1. Aged–Services for–United States. 2. Aged–Care–United States 3. Aged–United States–Psychology. 4. Apathy. I. O'Brien, James G.

HV1461 .S45 2000
362.6'0973-dc21
                                              00-021100

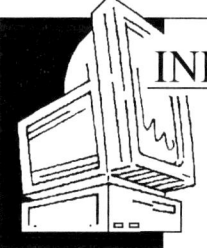

INDEXING & ABSTRACTING

Contributions to this publication are selectively indexed or abstracted in print, electronic, online, or CD-ROM version(s) of the reference tools and information services listed below. This list is current as of the copyright date of this publication. See the end of this section for additional notes.

- *Abstracts in Social Gerontology: Current Literature on Aging*
- *AgeInfo CD-Rom*
- *AgeLine Database*
- *Alzheimer's Disease Education & Referral Center (ADEAR)*
- *Behavioral Medicine Abstracts*
- *Brown University Geriatric Research Application Digest "Abstracts Section"*
- *BUBL Information Service. An Internet-based Information Service for the UK higher education community <URL:http://bubl.ac.uk/>*
- *Cambridge Scientific Abstracts*
- *caredata CD: the social & community care database*
- *CINAHL (Cumulative Index to Nursing & Allied Health Literature), in print, also on CD-ROM from CD PLUS, EBSCO, and SilverPlatter, and online from CDP Online (formerly BRS), Data-Star, and PaperChase. (Support materials include Subject Heading List, Database Search Guide, and instructional video)*
- *CNPIEC Reference Guide: Chinese National Directory of Foreign Periodicals*
- *Criminal Justice Abstracts*
- *Criminal Justice Periodical Index*
- *Current Contents: Clinical Medicine/Life Sciences (CC:CM/LS) (weekly Table of Contents Service), and Social Science Citation Index. Articles also searchable through Social SciSearch, ISI's online database and in ISI's Research Alert current awareness service*
- *Educational Administration Abstracts (EAA)*
- *Family Studies Database (online and CD/ROM)*
- *Family Violence & Sexual Assault Bulletin*
- *Human Resources Abstracts (HRA)*

(continued)

- *IBZ International Bibliography of Periodical Literature*
- *Index to Periodical Articles Related to Law*
- *MasterFILE: updated database from EBSCO Publishing*
- *Mental Health Abstracts (online through DIALOG)*
- *National Criminal Justice Reference Service*
- *New Literature on Old Age*
- *Sage Family Studies Abstracts (SFSA)*
- *Sage Urban Studies Abstracts (SUSA)*
- *Social Planning/Policy & Development Abstracts (SOPODA)*
- *Social Work Abstracts*
- *Sociological Abstracts (SA)*
- *Violence and Abuse Abstracts: A Review of Current Literature on Interpersonal Violence (VAA)*

Special Bibliographic Notes related to special journal issues (separates) and indexing/abstracting:

- indexing/abstracting services in this list will also cover material in any "separate" that is co-published simultaneously with Haworth's special thematic journal issue or DocuSerial. Indexing/abstracting usually covers material at the article/chapter level.
- monographic co-editions are intended for either non-subscribers or libraries which intend to purchase a second copy for their circulating collections.
- monographic co-editions are reported to all jobbers/wholesalers/approval plans. The source journal is listed as the "series" to assist the prevention of duplicate purchasing in the same manner utilized for books-in-series.
- to facilitate user/access services all indexing/abstracting services are encouraged to utilize the co-indexing entry note indicated at the bottom of the first page of each article/chapter/contribution.
- this is intended to assist a library user of any reference tool (whether print, electronic, online, or CD-ROM) to locate the monographic version if the library has purchased this version but not a subscription to the source journal.
- individual articles/chapters in any Haworth publication are also available through the Haworth Document Delivery Service (HDDS).

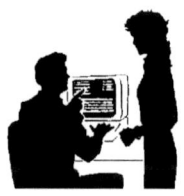

Self-Neglect:
Challenges
for Helping Professionals

Self-Neglect: Challenges for Helping Professionals has been co-published simultaneously as *Journal of Elder Abuse & Neglect*, Volume 11, Number 2 1999.

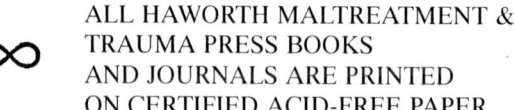

ALL HAWORTH MALTREATMENT & TRAUMA PRESS BOOKS AND JOURNALS ARE PRINTED ON CERTIFIED ACID-FREE PAPER

Self-Neglect: Challenges for Helping Professionals

CONTENTS

Preface–"Hector the Collector" *by Shel Silverstein*	xi

Self-Neglect: An Overview
   James G. O'Brien, MD
   Jane M. Thibault, PhD
   L. Carolyn Turner, MA
   Heather S. Laird-Fick, MD
	1

Indirect Life-Threatening Behavior in Elderly Patients
   Jane M. Thibault, PhD
   James G. O'Brien, MD
   L. Carolyn Turner, MA
	21

Ethics and Aging: Confronting Abuse and Self-Neglect
   Paul D. Simmons, PhD
   James G. O'Brien, MD
	33

Alcohol Abuse and Self-Neglect in the Elderly *Richard D. Blondell, MD*	55

Community Dimensions of Elderly Self-Neglect
   Mary Cay Sengstock, PhD, CCS
   Jane M. Thibault, PhD
   Rochelle Zaranek, MSW
	77

Index	95

Preface

HECTOR THE COLLECTOR

Hector the Collector
Collected bits of string,
Collected dolls with broken heads
And rusty bells that would not ring.
Pieces out of picture puzzles,
Bent-up nails and ice-cream sticks,
Twists of wires, worn-out tires,
Paper bags and broken bricks.

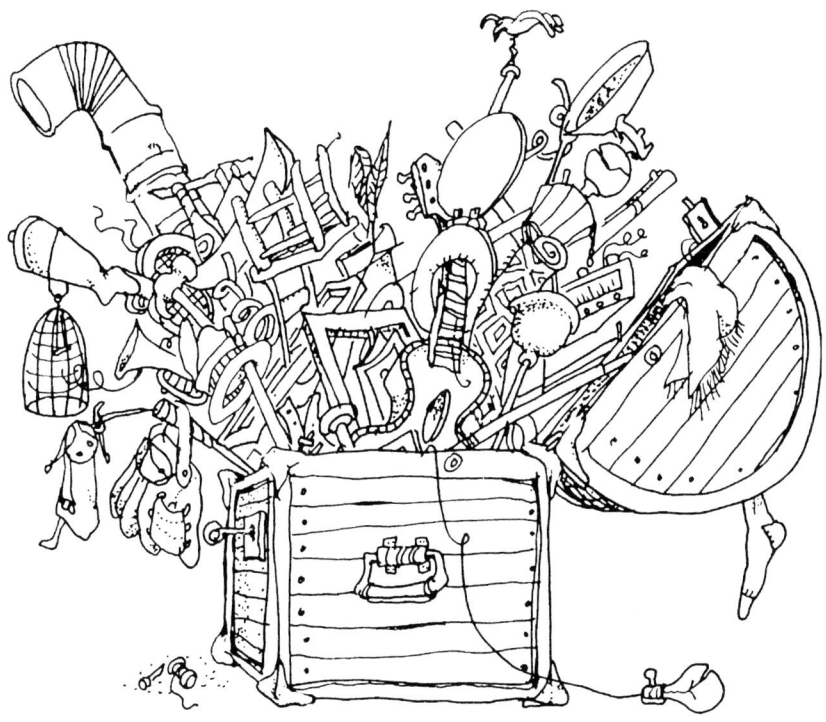

© 1974 *Where the Sidewalk Ends*. Printed with permission
HarperCollins *Publishers*

Old chipped vases, half shoelaces,
Gatlin' guns that wouldn't shoot,
Leaky boats that wouldn't float
And stopped-up horns that wouldn't toot.
Butter knives that had no handles,
Copper keys that fit no locks,
Rings that were too small for fingers,
Dried-up leaves and patched-up socks.
Worn-out belts that had no buckles,
'Lectric trains that had no tracks,
Airplane models, broken bottles,
Three-legged chairs and cups with cracks.
Hector the Collector
Loved these things with all his soul—
Loved them more than shining diamonds,
Loved them more than glistenin' gold.
Hector called to all the people,
"Come and share my treasure trunk!"
And all the silly sightless people
Came and looked . . . and called it junk.

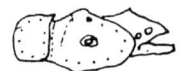

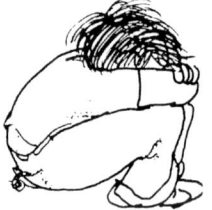

Self-Neglect:
An Overview

James G. O'Brien, MD
Jane M. Thibault, PhD
L. Carolyn Turner, MA
Heather S. Laird-Fick, MD

SUMMARY. Initially described in 1953, the concept of self-neglect is complex. Definitional problems exist because it can be redefined by changes in context. This article examines the epidemiology, etiology, detection, ethical/legal issues, management/intervention, and outcome. Prevention is particularly difficult given the nature of the problem, the poorly understood etiology, and the slow insidious progression of the syndrome before it reaches public attention. This complexity is compounded by the fact that respect for autonomy and personal rights is given paramount importance over paternalism when an intervention at an earlier stage could potentially result in a better outcome. *[Article copies available for a fee from The Haworth Document Delivery Service: 1-800-342-9678. E-mail address: getinfo@haworthpressinc.com <Website: http://www.haworthpressinc.com>]*

KEYWORDS. Self-neglect, autonomy, competency, recluse, Diogenes Syndrome

---

James G. O'Brien is Margaret D. Smock Endowed Chair and Professor, Division of Geriatrics, Department of Family and Community Medicine, University of Louisville School of Medicine, Louisville, KY 40292. Jane M. Thibault is Associate Professor, Division of Geriatrics, Department of Family and Community Medicine, University of Louisville School of Medicine. L. Carolyn Turner is Doctoral Candidate, Department of Psychology, Clinical Psychology Program, University of Louisville, Louisville, KY 40292. Heather S. Laird-Fick is affiliated with Academic Internal Medicine, 5333 McAuley Drive, Suuite 5011, Ypsilanti, MI 48197.

[Haworth co-indexing entry note]: "Self-Neglect: An Overview." O'Brien, James G. et al. Co-published simultaneously in *Journal of Elder Abuse & Neglect* (The Haworth Maltreatment & Trauma Press, an imprint of The Haworth Press, Inc.) Vol. 11, No. 2, 1999, pp. 1-19; and: *Self-Neglect: Challenges for Helping Professionals* (ed: James G. O'Brien) The Haworth Press, Inc., 1999, pp. 1-19. Single or multiple copies of this article are available for a fee from The Haworth Document Delivery Service [1-800-342-9678, 9:00 a.m. - 5:00 p.m. (EST). E-mail address: getinfo@haworthpressinc.com].

© 1999 by The Haworth Press, Inc. All rights reserved.

BACKGROUND

Self neglect as a phenomenon within the taxonomy of elder neglect and abuse has come of age. Erskine (1953) in his commentary on hermits and recluses initially described this phenomenon. Seven years later, Granick and Zeman (1960) published an exploratory study on the aged recluse. This was followed six years later by what seems to be the first article in the medical literature. Duncan MacMillan and Patricia Shaw described a syndrome of "senile breakdown" in the elderly in the *British Medical Journal* in 1966; subsequently, during the 1970s, a series of case reports and reviews appeared in various medical, psychiatric, and sociologic publications. Interest seemed to wane until more visibility was accorded in the late 1980s and early 1990s–particularly as a result of a national survey that identified self-neglect as the most frequently encountered form of elder abuse and neglect reported to state agencies (National Center for Elder Abuse [NCEA], 1998). Some view the inclusion of reports of self-abuse or neglect in state or national statistics on elder abuse and neglect as controversial. Yet these reports represent a large portion of victims served by Adult Protective Service (APS) agencies and thus include a large population with unmet needs (Lachs & Pillemer, 1995).

The concept of self-neglect is complex. Most individuals engage in some behavior or activity that could, in a broad sense, constitute self-neglect. Behaviors such as not being at ideal body weight, ingesting toxic substances (e.g., alcohol, smoking), not wearing seat belts, driving at excessive speeds, and not complying with medical recommendations are commonly encountered in the normal population. These activities are unlikely to result in any action either by a public authority, social service agency, or the courts. Clearly there is a threshold that needs to be exceeded before the label of self-neglect is attached.

Major definitional problems exist because self-neglect can be redefined by changes in context, such as the presence or absence of caregivers, cultural and community norms, the presence or absence of mental illness, the capacity to accept or refuse treatment. Furthermore, case reports and review articles dominate this literature, with a few notable exceptions (Baker, 1976; Clark, Mankikar, & Gray, 1975; Longres, 1994; MacMillan & Shaw, 1966; Radebaugh, Hooper, & Gruenberg, 1987; Wrigley & Cooney, 1992). Unfortunately, the definition of self-abuse varies from study to study and country to country, which makes interpreting this body of work more difficult.

The confusion over the definition is highlighted by the fact that the National Elder Abuse Incidence Study, (NCEA, 1998) excludes from its definition of self-neglect (and therefore from its incidence data) those situations in which a mentally competent older person, one who understands the consequences of his/her decisions, makes a conscious and voluntary decision to engage in acts that threaten his/her health or safety. This exclusion certainly is at odds with other studies of the phenomenon of elder self-neglect that have been described in the literature, particularly in the British literature. Baker and Miller (1991), Clark et al. (1975), MacMillan and Shaw (1966), and Radebaugh et al. (1987) in their studies included individuals who were cognitively intact and some of whom refused assistance.

MacMillan and Shaw, in their 1966 article on self-abuse, or "senile breakdown syndrome," have described a number of recluses, whose lack of personal hygiene was mirrored by the filth and dilapidation of their homes and perpetuated by their consistent refusal of assistance. The authors' definition of this syndrome included five characteristics of the victim and ten of the home. Victims were graded on a five-point scale with the most severe types being included in the study. Refusal of services was not a reason for exclusion but was encountered frequently. Since that article, self abuse has appeared sporadically in the literature under a variety of pseudonyms, including social breakdown syndrome, social breakdown in elderly, indirect self-destructive behavior, passive suicide, gross self-neglect, and Diogenes syndrome. In fact, Reed and Leonard (1989) have listed 20 different terms all related to self-neglect. Kastenbaum and Mishara (1971) noted self-injurious behavior in 44% of a hospitalized group of individuals over a 7-day period. Certainly this group represented one of the subtypes described by Reed and Leonard in the spectrum of self-neglecting elders.

Clark et al. (1975) coined the term "Diogenes Syndrome," which subsequently has been the favored terminology in Britain until recently when the name has been criticized as misleading. Patients with Diogenes syndrome have been described according to their "self-neglect, domestic squalor, social withdrawal, apathy, a tendency to hoard rubbish (syllogomania) and often a lack of shame" (Clark et al., 1975; Cybulska & Rucinski, 1986). These patients span the socioeconomic spectrum (Clark et al., 1975; Wrigley & Cooney, 1992).

In contrast to this widely accepted British characterization, early American researchers took more quantitative approaches (Gruenberg, Brandon, & Kasius, 1966) and dubbed the phenomenon "social breakdown syndrome" (SBS). Criteria for SBS include disruptive behavior and loss of function. This approach continues to be favored by organizations like the National Association of Adult Protective Services Administrators (NAAPSA), which defines self-neglect as:

> The result of an adult's inability, due to physical and/or mental impairments or diminished capacity, to perform essential self-care tasks including: providing essential food, clothing, shelter, and medical care; obtaining goods and services necessary to maintain physical health, mental health, emotional well-being and general safety; and/or managing financial affairs. (Duke, 1991, p. 27)

Others describe self-neglect in more healthcare-related terms and suggest that self-neglect refers to the physically ill individual who intentionally neglects prescribed self-care activities despite available resources and knowledge (Reed & Leonard, 1989). Under this definition, Diogenes syndrome would be excluded as an "illegitimate case" of self-neglect because it is not limited only to healthcare-related behaviors. The same researchers have conceptualized self-neglect as negative behavior that diminishes quality of life and thus warrants intervention. They also identify attributes necessary for a diagnosis of self-neglect:

1. The behavior has notable potential to be harmful or life threatening.
2. There is no specific purpose expressed or clearly identifiable reason for engaging in the behavior.
3. The behavior is not intended to end one's life immediately.
4. Effects of the behavior are cumulative and realized over time.
5. The behavior represents a repetitive pattern that provides several dimensions of self-care needs.

The qualitative and quantitative definitions are not mutually exclusive. Longres (1994), in examining self-neglect in Wisconsin, favors the NAAPSA definition, but nonetheless describes cases very much like those in the British literature. Other researchers have proposed more restrictive definitions.

In their 1992 report on a case of shared senile self-neglect between a married couple in their 60s, Cole, Gillet, and Fairburn have described the individuals as "domineering, quarrelsome, and independent." Such personality qualities are consistent with those in MacMillan and Shaw's (1966) original description of this condition, which they labeled "Senile Breakdown Syndrome." Another case study brings out an important facet often observed in these cases, specifically that the self-neglecting elder has not been an untidy person throughout his lifetime. In many cases, the self-neglect reflects a deterioration in adherence to formerly held standards of home and personal hygiene (Moore, 1989).

It would seem that the NAAPSA definition of self-neglect contains most of the critical elements of the syndrome, including failure to maintain acceptable levels of personal care, shelter, and health care. Individuals who appear to possess the capacity and refuse services should not be excluded from this definition.

EPIDEMIOLOGY

Epidemiologic characteristics can help health professionals identify who is at increased risk for self-neglect. Several studies have sought to delineate such risk factors; however, since the syndrome itself is so varied few truisms exist.

In the United States, self-neglect represents the most frequently reported form of elder abuse and neglect. One large study that gathered information from APS agencies and units on aging in all fifty states; Guam; Washington, DC; Puerto Rico; and the Virgin Islands (Tatara & Kuzmeskus, 1997), estimated the "prevalence" (total number of active cases during a one-year time period) of self-neglect cases to be 1.15 million and all other forms of elder abuse to be 1.10 million cases. The estimates of self-neglect were generated from data from only 30 states and then extrapolated to include all states. This estimate is open to challenge because the data were derived from only 30 states, a multiplier was used to estimate unreported cases, and the potential for duplication was not accounted for.

Another ambitious epidemiologic study that examined "incidence" (all new cases of abuse and neglect reported during a specified time period) of various forms of elder abuse and neglect reported that self-neglect represented roughly one in five of all cases of elder abuse/

neglect (NCEA, 1998). Significant differences between these two studies include the definitions of incidence vs. prevalence, which were used to guide data collection; the sampling methods used (in the NCEA study only 20 counties from 15 states were surveyed and appropriate estimations of national incidence rates were extrapolated from this 1996 data); and the statistical procedures from which annual estimations were made. This study also used sentinels in each community to independently identify victims. It was evident that data from APS agencies represented the "tip of the iceberg" with greater than five times that number going unreported and an additional group unknown and unidentified by sentinels.

In Wisconsin, self-neglect cases comprised 41.8% of all reported elder-abuse cases between 1986 and 1990 (Longres, 1994). MacMillan and Shaw (1966) and Wrigley and Cooney (1992) have reported rates of 0.5 per 1000 per year in England and Ireland, respectively. MacMillan and Shaw also have noted that the estimate of "pure" cases (removing patients with comorbid psychiatric diagnosis) was .23/1000. Their sampling methodology varied and these rates only represented referrals to psychiatric institutions; other patients may have sought help elsewhere or just not come to the attention of any authority or died without public attention. In addition, MacMillan and Shaw actively recruited participants for their study from a variety of referral sources in their community, which may have resulted in a higher incidence than might be expected. Furthermore, as the self-abuse literature reiterates, these individuals frequently have been recognized by community agencies long before they come to the attention of the medical profession, but apparently have not exceeded a threshold to precipitate intervention or have actively refused help from any formal authority.

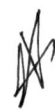

Self-abuse has been described primarily among older adults, particularly those over age 70 years (Longres, 1994; MacMillan & Shaw, 1966; Radebaugh et al., 1987; Tatara & Kuzmeskus, 1997; Wrigley & Cooney, 1992). In Tatara and Kuzmeskus's 1997 prevalence study using APS data with an age cut-off of 60 years, 63.6% of self-abusers were white; 57%, over age 75 years; and 64.2%, female. These data were consistent with findings in the NCEA incidence study. In the incidence study, 65.3% of the substantiated victims were female, and 65% were over age 75 years. Approximately 77.4% were white and 20.4% were black, which exceeds their representation in the general population. Seventy-five percent suffered from confusion with 34.3% incapable of caring for themselves. A number of authors have suggested that self-abusers tend to exhibit above-average intelligence (Cole et al., 1992). Clark et al. (1975) have reported that 15/30 patients demonstrated higher than average IQ. Women constitute the bulk of such patients in most studies, although men may be at higher risk (Longres, 1994; Radebaugh et al., 1987).

Most patients who engage in self-neglect live alone (Longres, 1994; MacMillan & Shaw, 1966; Wrigley & Cooney, 1992), although married couples (Cole et al., 1992; MacMillan & Shaw, 1966; Snowdon, 1987) and adults who live with others (Snowdon, 1987) have been identified. If the victim does reside with others, differentiating between self-neglect and elder neglect perpetrated by others may become problematic (Longres, 1994; O'Mahony & Evans, 1994). In fact, social isolation is an important criterion for self abuse (Longres, 1994; MacMillan & Shaw, 1966). The question becomes whether the isolation is self-imposed or situational. In some cases, it would appear to be actively sought despite regular contact with friends or relatives (Clark et al., 1975; Ungvari & Hantz, 1991; Wrigley & Cooney, 1992); whereas in others, the elderly express regret over their isolation (Longres, 1994).

Comorbidities, both physical and psychiatric, have received much attention. Early reports have described victims of self-neglect as having multiple physical aliments, and high rates of falls or other acute presentations with increased mortality (Baker, 1976; Clark et al., 1975; MacMillan & Shaw, 1966; Roe, 1977; Wrigley & Cooney, 1992). Loss of special senses, alcoholism, and memory impairment have been noted (MacMillan & Shaw, 1966; Roe, 1977; Snowdon, 1987). Compared with the general population, self-abusers are more likely to have dementia or to abuse alcohol (Longres, 1994; Radebaugh et al., 1987; Wrigley, 1992). Despite this increased risk, as many as half of self abusers will not have comorbid dementia or psychiatric diagnoses (Clark et al., 1975; MacMillan & Shaw, 1966; Radebaugh et al., 1987; Wrigley & Cooney, 1992). Gruenberg et al. (1987) have noted that 68% of those with SBS had no identifiable comorbid mental illness. Roe (1977) also has noted that the majority of victims admitted to his unit experienced a significant improvement in quality of life.

Most of the research thus far profiles the typical victim of self-neglect to be female, older, living in isolation and in squalor, with significant co-morbid conditions such as a mental illness or alcoholism, but often functionally capable.

ETIOLOGY

A clear concept of the etiology of self-neglect is more elusive than its epidemiology. This occurs for a variety of reasons not the least of which is that the studies thus far have not used consistent methodology or definitions and typically focus on a small number of cases making it more difficult to search for causes of self-neglect. Studies from various countries, cultures, and different systems of care contribute to the lack of consensus on definition. In addition, self-abuse as a syndrome may include a broad spectrum of etiologic factors making it impossible to identify any single precipitating event or cause. This is certainly consistent with other syndromes encountered in geriatric medicine.

Several theories about the etiology have been proposed. MacMillan and Shaw (1966) have suggested that a pre-syndrome personality predisposes one to the development of self-neglect based on their study of the pre-morbid personality of 72 patients assessed over a three-year period. Information was derived from the referring source; home visits; and interviews with relatives, neighbors, friends, their general practitioner, and social worker. A pattern that emerged was of a domineering, quarrelsome, and independent individual who was often described as independent, unfriendly, stubborn, obstinate, aloof, aggressive, suspicious, secretive, and quarrelsome. These characteristics seem to hold for a pre-morbid personality type whether the individuals were "mentally normal" or were psychotic.

A pattern of gradual withdrawal from the community and a rejection of services also seemed to emerge. Many of these individuals were well known to social agencies and local authorities well in advance of being labeled as self-neglect victims requiring intervention (Wrigley & Cooney, 1992). Baker (1976) has described a slowly progressive syndrome with multiple co-morbidities and progressive dementia ultimately resulting in some crisis forcing outside intervention and subsequent institutionalization. So there may be a long prodrome to this syndrome.

Clark et al. (1975) also noted pre-morbid characteristics such as being aloof, detached, shrewd, suspicious, and less well-integrated;

less significant traits included being less stable, emotionally more serious, aggressive, and group-dependent with a tendency to distort reality. They also noted that many individuals had a high IQ and had been successful in their former lives. MacMillan and Shaw (1966) completed a psychometric evaluation on 28 of the 72 patients and found not one instance of mental sub-normality. Twenty-five percent were in the high-average intelligence.

Whitehead (1975) has suggested that self-neglect reflects an exaggeration of life long standards of poor home and personal hygiene, this deterioration being brought on by the functional impairments of old age. Clark et al. (1975) have described a similar explanation: Individuals who give personal and domestic care a low priority resulting in a disorganized style of life that becomes exaggerated by aging and physical infirmity. They also posited that the syndrome might represent a reaction to stress in an elderly person with certain personality characteristics. Post (1982) in questioning the idea of an at risk personality, has noted, "personality structure does not break down on account of aging alone or without physical deterioration, especially of the brain. However, the personality with which the person enters late life will not only make him more or less vulnerable to functional psychiatric disorders, but will also determine their form and content."

Ungvari and Hantz (1991) have suggested that self-neglect might represent an atypical adjustment disorder superimposed on long-standing personality abnormalities including paranoid or schizoid traits. Precipitating events might include the loss of a loved one or some other stressful event. The overall picture of pure senile breakdown of the elderly (SBE) represents a distorted exaggeration of dissatisfaction, bitterness, and misanthropy sometimes associated with the psychology of old age. Social isolation and lack of confidants are not the cause of pure SBE but the consequence of the usually life-long personality problems.

The "diathesis-stress model of mental illness" (Meehl, 1962) may offer a workable model for the etiology of self-neglect. This model suggests that in response to particular stressors a person with a pre-existing vulnerability resulting from a personality disorder or a problematic personality will develop a mental illness. Thus the "at-risk personality" may respond differently and less adaptively to the same stressors with which all aging people are confronted, such as loss of a loved one, relocation, retirement, or increasing infirmity. MacMillan and Shaw (1966) have noted that the death of a spouse was the precipitant in 11 of 72 cases and also a complete absence of social support was noted in 8 of 72 in the same study. Increased rates of depression have been noted by Thompson, Gallager, and Czirr (1988). Changes in neurotransmission were felt to be the predisposing cause according to Cloninger (1987) and Pies and Popli (1995). The latter also implicated some abnormality in the serotonergic system in the pathophysiology of self-injurious behavior and other related behaviors. The population studied differed from the typical self-neglecting elder in the community because of definitional differences; the diversity in age; and the inclusion of mentally retarded individuals, autistic patients, prisoners, and psychiatric patients.

Other psychiatric diagnoses may present with or mimic self-abuse. Individuals with an obsessive-compulsive disorder may hoard and initially express shame over their behavior; whereas, the self-abusers typically lack any purpose to the hoarding (Greenberg & Witzum, 1990). Patients with schizophrenia, paranoia, organic mental disorders, or long standing alcohol abuse may also hoard or display self-neglecting behavior (Greenberg & Witzum, 1990; Post, 1982; Thibault & Maly, 1993). Baker and Miller (1991) have studied residents in a nursing home who withdrew from other residents and staff by engaging in a process of increasing isolation that the authors labeled as cocooning. This may represent the institutional equivalent of isolation in the community; in the institutional setting, however, residents are not allowed to deteriorate in terms of hygiene and self-care. Many of these individuals were diagnosed with depression and responded well to treatment.

Neuropsychiatric disorders have been proposed as a possible etiology. Dementia of the frontal lobe type certainly has been noted to mimic features of self-abuse with resulting neglect of personal hygiene, social break-down and personality change with lack of concern, loss of initiative and insight with paranoid symptoms (Orell, Sahakian, & Bergmann, 1991; Pies & Popli, 1995).

Another possible explanation is that self-neglect reflects an active expression of resentment or withdrawal from the community (MacMillan & Shaw, 1966). Thibault (1984) has proposed the concept of self-neglect as an active effort on the part of the individual to regain autonomy and control over his/her own circumstances and choices.

Self-neglect may also be conceptualized as an indirect suicidal behavior. Farberow (1980) and Reed and Leonard (1989) have supported a hypothesis such as this and have gone on to suggest that noncompliance is an indirect form of suicide. Given the degree of confusion over the etiology of the spectrum of behaviors encountered under the rubric of self-neglect clearly there is an established need for additional research in this area using larger populations.

DETECTION

Identifying victims of self-neglect in the community is a challenging task. Because of the nature of the problem these victims are likely to be isolated and unlikely to be in contact with the medical establishment; they may even be unnoticed in their own neighborhoods. If they are without family or a social network, the likelihood of anyone gaining access to the home to detect the problem is minimal. Neighbors and others in the area, including healthcare providers, may feel that the privacy of the individual and the family is of paramount importance and that one should not intervene without invitation. Access may be prohibited as a result of fear of being "put away" into an institution on the victim's part (MacMillan, 1969). Another barrier to detection and intervention noted by MacMillan and Shaw (1966) is the eccentricity of the behavior that may frighten neighbors or family members who otherwise might have helped.

Frequently these individuals come to the attention of an authority as a result of some dramatic decline in function often precipitated by an acute medical illness, such as falls, weakness, pneumonia, or stroke resulting in hospitalization (Clark et al., 1975; MacMillan, 1969; Roe, 1977). Although the phenomenon is recognized in most states, it is evident that many adult protective agencies would not intervene if the individual is determined to have the capacity to manage his own affairs and refuses services or assistance. Many victims may be known to social services agencies for years (Baker, 1976; Clark et al., 1975; Cole et al., 1992; MacMillan & Shaw, 1966; Wrigley & Cooney, 1992). Perhaps there should be an opportunity to intervene at an earlier stage, such as establishing at-risk registers to identify potential victims (Wrigley & Cooney, 1992). Balancing safety with patient autonomy is likely to present problems for earlier intervention.

ETHICAL/LEGAL ISSUES

Responding to a victim of self-neglect often results in the forced interface of social, medical, and legal services that are not as well coordinated in the United States as in other countries. Although reporting laws exist in all states, the definition of elder abuse and neglect and the specific reporting requirements are different in each state (Benton & Marshall, 1991; Brewer & Jones, 1989; Macolini, 1995; Thobaben & Anderson, 1985). Many, but not all, states specifically include self-neglect in their statutes about reporting, defining elder self-neglect as a person's failure to provide for the necessities of his or her own life (Lachs & Pillemer, 1995; Kapp, 1995). With regard to reporting elder abuse, elder-neglect, and elder self-neglect, there is no federal policy, but rather, "50 variations on a theme" (Thobaben & Anderson, 1985, p. 371).

Penalties for failure to report vary as well. In some states fines up to $1000 can be levied and sentences of a maximum of six months imprisonment can be imposed. Some states include licensing sanctions as potential punishment for failure to report; also, some states penalize non-reporting practitioners by awarding damages to the victim from the time that the practitioner was aware of the abuse/neglect (Brewer & Jones, 1989).

Most states require healthcare providers and others to report suspected self-neglect to appropriate agencies. By law, patients are afforded the right to refuse intervention or treatment as long as they are deemed competent to make these decisions (Benton & Marshall, 1991) and their behavior does not jeopardize the rights/health of others.

Capacity to decide is a legal determination but typically the evaluation is performed by health care providers. The individual must understand the information, must not be under duress, and must be able to articulate the choices and consequences of that decision. Further, the decision must be consistent with the individual's values.

The right to self-determination is ethically and legally compromised, however, when an individual is suffering from depression, dementia, or other conditions that diminish his/her capacity for rationality–comprehending information and making informed decisions. Before practitioners can simply respect the patient's right to autonomy and his/her decision to refuse treatment, they must determine that the patient is competent to make decisions and that these decisions are in fact informed and voluntary (Cutler & Tisdale, 1992). Legal interventions are of importance in the cases of self-neglect on the part of individuals who are incapable of making appropriate decisions. When a self-neglecting elder is determined incompetent by the court or competent but jeopardizing the rights and health of others, possible legal interventions include involuntary commitment, appointment of a guardian, or court-ordered adult protective services including homemaking and in-home nursing.

MANAGEMENT/INTERVENTION

The literature provides little help in terms of model programs to manage self-neglect. In-patient behavioral modification in conjunction with the use of medications such as antidepressants to treat underlying problems such as depression has been demonstrated to show success in isolated cases (Ungvari & Hantz, 1991). Nursing approaches such as Orem's self-care model have been suggested (Moore, 1989), whereas care teams and at-risk registries in Ireland have been initiated (Wrigley & Cooney, 1992). Repeated attempts to get self-abusers to participate in day-care hospitals have met with mixed results. These patients often resume hoarding after their homes have been cleaned or simply refuse assistance necessitating persistence and patience on the part of caretakers.

Such refusals, a hallmark of self-abuse, pose an ethical and medicolegal dilemma for health care professionals. Twenty-eight states currently recognize self abuse, either legally or administratively (Longres, 1994). However, the prevailing concept of patient autonomy empowers competent individuals to accept or refuse medical interventions. Since approximately half of all patients who neglect themselves have no underlying mental illnesses, they are well within their rights in refusing treatment. Most authors appear comfortable with these situations (Clark et al., 1975; Henderson-Smith, 1975; MacAnespie, 1975; Roe, 1977). Henderson-Smith (1975) went so far as to write: "That some independently minded old people resist the pressure of society to conform should be a source of satisfaction to those who care for the freedom of the human spirit" (p. 55).

Other British authors support intervention despite patient refusal, citing the risks of fire, vermin, and spread of disease associated with hoarding and uncleanliness (Shah, 1992; Thomasma, 1984; Twomey, 1975). They have suggested taking public health action under the auspices of local authorities or national laws. MacMillan (1969) has recommended integrated services including social, medical, psychiatric, and community services given the comprehensive needs of such individuals.

The philosophy underlying management should be that each person is treated as an individual and respect paid to his wishes. Henderson-Smith (1975), Roe (1977), and Wrigley and Cooney (1992) have suggested hospitalization as a means of intervention with the potential for a good outcome. Clearly this is in contrast with the views of Clark et al. (1975) who have noted the poor outcome with a high mortality rate in their post-hospitalization study. Additionally they have recommended respecting the rights and opinions of victims even if they choose to live in squalor.

MacMillan and Shaw (1966) have noted the valuable roles of day care, home-help, home-nursing, and health visitor services. Baker (1976) has questioned the benefit to the victim even if life is extended as the result of an intervention with medical and nursing care. Longres (1994) has highlighted the problems for practitioners, "for they must deal effectively with the contradictions involved in it: namely that rights for autonomy, independence, and self-determination must be balanced against the need to build community and show concern for the welfare of others" (p. 6).

One of the case workers in the Longres study showing great insight and sensitivity has suggested to approach the victim by playing "to their sense of isolation, their sense of their history, who they are, who they were when they were younger and who they are now. If we keep that in perspective and the values that these people have, that they can still contribute" (p. 12). Wrigley and Cooney (1992) have recommended individualizing care. A recent report by Dyer et al. (1999) attests to the value of incorporating APS workers into geriatric assessment teams to address the problems of abuse and neglect.

An approach that imposes the least restrictive solution on the victim, while attempting to balance safety and autonomy, is imperative. When the actions of the victim are putting others at risk, however, a paternalistic approach is warranted. Given that victims are more likely to view offers of help as being intrusive (Longres, 1994), sensitivity and gentle persistence are more likely to be associated with a positive outcome for the victim.

OUTCOME

The outcome for individuals who engage in self-neglect is not well established. MacMillan and Shaw (1966) in their original study have noted that some patients deteriorated after admission to the hospital and that the majority rapidly deteriorated with very few living in the community after three years. They reported a mortality rate of 50% over 4 years–a rate that affected women to an inordinate degree. Baker in 1976 painted an even bleaker picture. He noted that 25% of self-neglecting elders died in the first 3 weeks after admission, and that soon after admission patients became bewildered, restless, and unable to report on their needs except express a desire to go home. He also noted an increased prevalence of apathy, diminished appetite, and onset of incontinence and an increase in the frequency of falls. Clark et al. (1975) have noted that in patients admitted to a hospital with a diagnosis of self-abuse, the mortality rate was excessively high especially for women who experienced a 46% mortality rate. Patients tended to present in crisis with multiple diagnoses including heart failure, stroke, and pneumonia. Roe (1977) has reported 12% mortality within three weeks of admission and a long-term inpatient expected mortality of 36%. He has also noted, however, that 60% of these patients had a better quality of life after admission. Wrigley and Cooney (1992) in a Dublin study found that within a two-year period 41% of patients admitted to an inpatient psychiatric unit returned home, 34% were in continuing care in nursing homes, and 18% had died.

Wrigley and Cooney (1992) in their study discovered 29 individuals with Diogenes Syndrome with 2/3 having significant co-morbidities such as senile dementia, alcoholism, and schizophrenia likely to result in a more rapid decline with a reported mortality rate of 18%. Lachs et al. (1998) in a cohort study of all individuals referred to Adult Protective Services in New Haven noted a marked increase in mortality for those identified as victims of self-neglect–an 83% mortality rate after 13 years. Victims of abuse by others had an even higher mortality rate–91%. The average age of the cohort at the inception of the study was 74 years.

It is difficult to form an opinion or prognosis from the available data. Some studies consisted of a retrospective review of hospital records and did not involve random or stratified sampling. The number of subjects in most studies was small. Participants sometimes were actively recruited (MacMillan & Shaw, 1966). Others were identified from patients referred to psychiatric units (Clark et al., 1975; Wrigley & Cooney, 1992) or geriatric units (Baker, 1976). Some studies looked at data derived from reports to state APS agencies (Longres, 1994; NCEA, 1998; Tatara & Kuzmeskus, 1997).

PREVENTION

Prevention of elder neglect is particularly difficult given the complex nature of the problem, the poorly understood etiology, and the slow insidious progression of the syndrome before it reaches public attention. This complexity is compounded by the fact that respect for autonomy and personal rights are given paramount importance over paternalism when an intervention at an earlier stage could potentially result in a better outcome.

Given the etiologic possibility of a pre-morbid personality preceding the self-neglect, this behavior may or may not be amenable to modification. Longres in his 1994 study profiling the self-neglecting elder has noted frequent problems with mental illness, dementia, alcohol and drug problems–potentially treatable diseases that with appropriate intervention could prevent progression to a full blown syndrome. Wrigley and Cooney (1992) in their study have noted that 79% of the victims were known to public health nurses prior to referral and that many of these people were tolerated by neighbors for years prior to intervention. This certainly is consistent with many other studies and suggests that there may be a potential for secondary or tertiary prevention at that stage. MacMillan (1969) has identified the important role of the general practitioner in the community who is likely to encounter patients at a much earlier stage of the breakdown. He goes on to suggest practical measures for the prevention of senile breakdown such as integrating hospital and community services and establishing full liaison between geriatric and psychogeriatric services. He also points to the need for enhanced communication, the development of joint domiciliary visitation, day centers, day hospitals, short-term inpatient admissions, and a joint assessment unit. Although these recommendations were made more than 30 years ago in a different country, they have definite application in contemporary American society. Disconnected health-care, social, and mental health services and the court system compound the detection, management, and prevention of this problem today.

REFERENCES

Baker, A. (1976). Slow euthanasia–or 'she will be better off in hospital.' *British Medical Journal, 2*, 571-572.
Baker, F., & Miller, C. (1991). 'Cocooning': A clinical sign of geriatric depression in geriatric patients. *Hospital and Community Psychiatry, 42*, 845-846.
Benton, D., & Marshall, C. (1991). Elder abuse. *Clinics in Geriatric Medicine, 7*, 831-845.
Berlyne, N. (1975). Diogenes syndrome [letter]. *Lancet, i*(7909), 515.
Brewer, R., & Jones, J. (1989). Reporting elder abuse: Limitations of statutes. *Annals of Emergency Medicine, 18*, 1277-1221.
Clark, A., Mankikar, G., & Gray, I. (1975). Diogenese syndrome: A clinical study of gross self-neglect in old age. *Lancet, i*(7903), 366-368.
Cole, A., Gillett, T., & Fairburn, A. (1992). A case of senile self-neglect in a married couple: 'Diogenese a deux'? *International Journal of Geriatric Psychiatry, 7*, 839-841.
Cloninger, C. (1987). A systematic method for clinical description and classification of personality variants. *Archives of General Psychiatry, 44*, 573-578.
Cutler, S., & Tisdale, W. (1992). Ethical issues in working with self-neglect. In E. Rathbone-McCuan & R. Fabian (Eds.), *Self-Neglecting Elders* (pp. 27-45). New York: Auburn House.
Cybulska, E., & Rucinski, J. (1986). Gross self-neglect in old age. *British Journal of Hospital Medicine, 36*, 21-25.
Duke, J. (1991). A national study of self-neglecting APS clients. In T. Tatara & M. Rittman (Eds.), Koffer-Flores, K. (Coordinator) *Findings of five elder abuse studies* (pp. 23-53). Washington, DC: National Aging Resource Center on Elder Abuse.
Dyer, C., Gleason, M., Murphy, K., Paveik, V., Partal, B., Regev, T., & Hyman, D. (1999). Treating elder neglect: Collaboration between a geriatrics assessment team and adult protective services. *Southern Medical Journal, 92*, 242-244.
Erksine, H. (1953). *Out of this world–A collection of hermits and recluses*. New York: Putnam.
Farberow, N. (1980). *The many faces of suicide: Indirect self-destructive behavior*. New York: McGraw-Hill.
Gannon, M., & O'Boyle, J. (1992). Diogenese syndrome. [editorial]. *Irish Medical Journal, 85*, 124.
Granick, R., & Zeman, F. (1960). The aged recluse–An exploratory study with particular reference to community responsibility. *Journal of Chronic Disease, 12*, 639-653.
Greenberg, D., & Witzum, A. (1990). Hoarding as a psychiatric symptom. *Journal of Clinical Psychiatry, 51*, 417-421.

Gruenberg, E., Brandon, S., & Kasius, R. (1966). Identifying cases of the social breakdown syndrome. In E. Greunger (Ed.), *Evaluating the effectiveness of community mental health services* (pp. 127-143). New York: Millbank Memorial Fund.

Henderson-Smith, S. (1975). Diogenes syndrome. [letter]. *Lancet, i*(7909), 515.

Hogstell, M. (1993). Understanding hoarding behaviors in the elderly. *American Journal of Nursing, 93*(7), 42-45.

Kapp, J. (1995). Elder mistreatment: Legal interventions and policy uncertainties. *Behavioral Sciences and the Law, 13*, 365-389.

Kastenbaum, R., & Mishara, B. (1971). Premature death and self-injurious behavior in old age. *Geriatrics, 26*, 71-81.

Lachs, M., & Pillemer, K. (1995). Current concepts: Abuse and neglect of elderly persons. *The New England Journal of Medicine, 332*, 437-443.

Lachs, M., Williams, C., O'Brien, S., Pillemer, K., & Charlson, M. (1998). The mortality of elder mistreatment. *The Journal of the American Medical Association, 280*, 428-432.

Longres, F. (1994). Self-neglect and social control: A modest test of an issue. *Journal of Gerontological Social Work, 22*, 3-20.

MacAnespie, H. (1975). Diogenes syndrome. [letter]. *Lancet, i*(7909), 750.

MacMillan, D., (1969). Features of senile breakdown. *Geriatrics, 24*, 109-118.

MacMillan, D. & Shaw, P. (1966). Senile breakdown in standards of personal and environmental cleanliness. *British Medical Journal, 2*, 227-229.

Macolini, R. (1995). Elder abuse policy: Considerations in research and legislation. *Behavioral Sciences and the Law, 13*, 349-363.

Meehl, P. (1962). Schizotaxia, schizotypy, and schizophrenia. *American Psychologist, 17*, 827-838.

Ming Chan, K., & Beard, K. (1993). A patient with recurrent hypothermia with thrombocytopenia. *Postgraduate Medical Journal, 69*, 227-229.

Moore, R. (1989). Diogenes syndrome. *Nursing Times, 85*, 46-48.

National Center on Elder Abuse (NCEA) at the American Public Human Services Association. (1998). *National Elder Abuse Study: Final report.* Washington, DC: Author.

O'Mahony, D., & Evans, J. (1994). Diogenes syndrome by proxy. *British Journal of Psychiatry, 164*, 705-706.

Orrell, M., Sahakian, B., & Bergmann, K. (1989). Self-neglect and frontal lobe dysfunction. *British Journal of Psychiatry, 155*, 101-105.

Orrell, M., & Sahakian, B. (1991). Dementia of the frontal lobe type. *Psychological Medicine, 212*, 553-556.

Pies, R., & Popli, A. (1995). Self-injurious behavior: Pathophysiology and implications for treatment. *Journal of Clinical Psychiatry, 56*, 580-588.

Post, F. (1982). Functional disorders I. Description, incidence, and recognition. In R. Levy & F. Post, (Eds.), *In the psychiatry of late life* (pp. 176-196). Oxford: Blackwell Scientific.

Radebaugh, T., Hooper, F., & Gruenberg, E. (1987). The social breakdown syndrome in the elderly population living in the community: The helping study. *British Journal of Psychiatry, 151*, 341-346.

Reed, P., & Leonard, V. (1989). An analysis of the concept of self-neglect. *Advanced Nursing Science, 12*, 39-53.

Roe, P. (1977). Self-neglect. *Age and Aging, 6*, 192-194.

Shah, A. (1992). Self-neglect in adult life. [letter; comment]. *British Journal of Psychiatry, 161*, 865.

Snowdon, J. (1987). Uncleanliness among persons seen by community health workers. *Hospital and Community Psychiatry, 38*, 491-494.

Tantam, D. (1988). Lifelong eccentricity and social isolation, I. Psychiatric social and forensic aspects. *British Journal of Psychiatry, 153*, 777-782.

Tatara, T., & Kuzmeskus, L. (1997). *Summaries of the statistical data on elder abuse in domestic settings for FY 95 and FY 96.* Washington, DC: National Center on Elder Abuse.

Thibault, J. (1984). *The analysis and treatment of indirect self-destructive behaviors in the elderly.* Unpublished doctoral dissertation, University of Chicago, Chicago.

Thibault, J., & Maly, R. (1993). Recognition and treatment of substance abuse in the elderly. *Primary Care; Clinics in Office Practice, 20*, 155-165.

Thobaben, M., & Anderson, L. (1985). The legal side. Reporting elder abuse: It's the law. *The American Journal of Nursing, 85*, 371-374.

Thomasma, D. (1984). Freedom, dependency and the care of the very old. *Journal of the American Geriatric Society, 32*, 906-914.

Thompson, L., Gallager, D., & Czirr, R. (1988). Personality disorders and outcome in the treatment of late-life depression. *Journal of Geriatric Psychiatry, 21*, 133-153.

Twomey, J. (1975). Diogenes syndrome. [letter]. *Lancet, i*(7909), 515.

Ungvari, G., & Hantz, P. (1991). Social breakdown in the elderly, II. Sociodemographic data and psychopathology. *Comprehensive Psychiatry, 32*, 445-449.

Vostanis, P., & Dean, C. (1992). Self-neglect in adult life. *British Journal of Psychiatry, 161*, 265-267.

Whitehead, T. (1975). Diogenes syndrome. [letter]. *Lancet, i*(7909), 628.

Williams-Burgess, C., & Kimball, M. (1992). The neglected elder: A family systems approach. *Journal of Psychosocial Nursing and Mental Health Services, 30*, 21-25.

Wrigley, M., & Cooney, C. (1992). Diogenes syndrome–An Irish series. *Irish Journal of Psychological Medicine, 9*, 37-41.

Indirect Life-Threatening Behavior in Elderly Patients

Jane M. Thibault, PhD
James G. O'Brien, MD
L. Carolyn Turner, MA

SUMMARY. Older adults frequently engage in such indirect life-threatening behaviors as extreme lack of self-care, refusal to eat, refusal to take medications, and failure to comply with an understood medical regimen. These behaviors are often classified as non-compliance or passive suicide. Analysis of such phenomena reveals that these actions can represent attempts by the person to gain control of and to ameliorate a negative life situation. A case is presented which demonstrates the ultimate outcome of engagement in such behavior when it is misinterpreted and left untreated. The functions of indirect life-threatening behavior are discussed. *[Article copies available for a fee from The Haworth Document Delivery Service: 1-800-342-9678. E-mail address: getinfo@haworthpressinc.com <Website: http://www.haworthpressinc.com>]*

KEYWORDS. Self-neglect, passive suicide, non-compliance, personal control

---

Jane M. Thibault is Associate Professor, Division of Geriatrics, Department of Family and Community Medicine, University of Louisville School of Medicine, Louisville, KY 40292. James G. O'Brien is Margaret D. Smock Endowed Chair and Professor, Division of Geriatrics, Department of Family and Community Medicine, University of Louisville School of Medicine, Louisville, KY 40292. L. Carolyn Turner is Doctoral Candidate, Department of Psychology, Clinical Psychology Program, University of Louisville, Louisville, KY 40292.

[Haworth co-indexing entry note]: "Indirect Life-Threatening Behavior in Elderly Patients." Thibault, Jane M., James G. O'Brien, and L. Carolyn Turner. Co-published simultaneously in *Journal of Elder Abuse & Neglect* (The Haworth Maltreatment & Trauma Press, an imprint of The Haworth Press, Inc.) Vol. 11, No. 2, 1999, pp. 21-32; and: *Self-Neglect: Challenges for Helping Professionals* (ed: James G. O'Brien) The Haworth Press, Inc., 1999, pp. 21-32. Single or multiple copies of this article are available for a fee from The Haworth Document Delivery Service [1-800-342-9678, 9:00 a.m. - 5:00 p.m. (EST). E-mail address: getinfo@haworthpressinc.com].

© 1999 by The Haworth Press, Inc. All rights reserved.

INTRODUCTION

Health care providers deal not only with the duty to maintain health and forestall death, but also with the task of preserving the "human integrity" of their patients and clients (Kastenbaum & Mishara, 1971). These duties can become complicated when patients engage in life-threatening behavior patterns. In addition to overtly suicidal behavior and direct life-threatening actions (such as shooting oneself, cutting oneself with a knife, or taking an overdose of medication), providers are also aware of more subtle behaviors on the part of patients that often lead to premature death. Such indirect life-threatening behavior is recognized as having a delayed, insidious effect on health but is often overlooked or misinterpreted by family members, caregivers, and health care providers. Unfortunately, many patients die because of indirect life-threatening behavior, which hastens death with or without the conscious intent to commit self-harm on the part of the patient.

Treatment of older adults in ambulatory, tertiary, and long-term care settings reveals the frequent occurrence of indirect life-threatening behavior (ILTB) in this client population. ILTB includes such actions as extreme self-neglect, refusal to eat or drink, refusal to take prescribed medications, and failure to comply with an understood medical regimen. The incidence of ILTB in the general elderly population is not specifically known. To date, relatively few researchers have examined the incidence and associated features of ILTB, perhaps because of the difficulty in developing a unified theory of the etiology of this complex phenomenon.

REVIEW OF THE LITERATURE

The operational difference between direct self-destructive behavior, or suicide, and indirect life-threatening behavior is described by Nelson and Farberow, two early investigators of this phenomenon. They make the following distinction:

> Direct self-destructive behavior, or suicide, implies active participation in a life-threatening act through which one willfully intends to take one's own life. . . Indirect life-threatening behavior does not usually involve the initiation of a life-threatening act that is likely to prove fatal as a direct and immediate consequence

of the act itself. . . The relationship between direct and indirect self-destructive behavior is also poorly understood, that is, whether they are part of the same continuum or are arranged in different conceptual spheres. (Nelson & Farberow, 1977, p. 125)

The authors also state that "While the impact of overt suicidal behavior has been much researched, little is known of the death that has been prematurely hastened through the use of indirect self-destructive activity" (p. 125).

There are several other terms that are often substituted for indirect self-destructive behavior. These include "hidden suicide" (Meerloo, 1968), "subintentional suicide" (Schneidman, 1968), "alternative suicide" and "suicidal equivalent." Menninger (1938) uses the terms "partial suicide" and "focal suicide," which appear to convey the same meaning as indirect life-threatening behavior. He assigns behaviors such as martyrdom, asceticism, self-mutilation, malingering, repeated surgeries, alcoholism, addictions, and hypochondriasis to this category. Nelson and Farberow originally used the term "indirect life-threatening behavior" in 1977; Farberow changed the term to "indirect self-destructive behavior" in 1980. Both of these terms are more general and include a greater variety of behaviors than the terms using the word "suicide." A recent but more behaviorally specific term used by Rathbone-McCuan and Fabian (1992) and others is "self-neglect." In summary, Nelson and Farberow state that indirect self-destructive behavior "may injure, defeat, distress, and shorten life as much as direct self-destructive behavior," but "while its occurrence has been clinically apparent for some time, it has remained unclear and as yet not systematically explored" (p. 127).

Early research examined self-destructive behavior patterns and their associated personality characteristics and psychosocial variables in chronically and terminally ill patients. The first investigators, Duncan MacMillan and Patricia Shaw, described the phenomenon as "senile breakdown" in their study of a small group of patients who had ceased maintaining local standards of cleanliness and hygiene (MacMillan & Shaw, 1966). In a study of elderly chronically ill patients, Nelson and Farberow (1997) found that those most likely to engage in ILTB had experienced significantly more personal losses, expressed more dissatisfaction with their medical care, and were rated as more manipulative and risk-taking than patients not performing ILTB. Diabetic patients who were noncompliant with medical treatment were observed to be lower in frustration tolerance and the ability to delay gratification, and more dependent and aggressive behaviorally than compliant patients (Farberow, Stein, Darbourne, & Hirsch, 1970). Similar findings were observed in a comparison of cooperative and non-cooperative Buerger's disease patients. Non-cooperative patients were perceived by providers to be more hostile, complaining, negativistic and manipulative than cooperative patients (Farberow & Nehemkis, 1979). In addition, these investigators found that non-cooperative patients did not place as much value on achievement, were more present- than future-oriented, and experienced the passage of time more slowly. Gerber and colleagues (1981) studied the psychological and psychosocial features that discriminated between compliant and non-compliant chronically ill dialysis patients. The results of this analysis suggested that patients who harmed themselves indirectly through noncompliance with medical treatment experienced more subjective feelings of powerlessness and nervousness; felt less valued and appreciated by significant others; suffered greater blows to self-worth as a result of their illness; and were described as more irritable, suspicious, and dogmatic than their compliant cohorts.

Reed and Leonard (1989) analyzed the literature related to self-neglect and developed a concept of the etiology of the behavior, which she defined as "a pattern of intentionally neglecting prescribed self-care activities despite available resources and knowledge." Longres (1994) investigated the conflict between the patient's right to self-determination and the duty of the larger community to express concern for elders at health risk due to their self-neglectful behavior. He raised the question central to all intervention, "Where does self-determination and self-neglect begin?"

Most recently the Gruman, Stern, and Caro comparison of self-neglect and abuse in an elderly population indicated that those engaging in self-neglect had higher levels of impairment than did abused elders (1997).

CONCEPTUALIZATION OF ILTB

Understanding the person's motivation to engage in indirect life-threatening behavior is a challenge to the researcher and the practitioner alike. This syndrome of behaviors has multiple causes and each case must be examined closely to comprehend the meaning of the behavior for the specific patient. Failure to consider various explanations may result in ineffective interventions. Analysis of the sparse and very varied literature dealing with the phenomenon reveals the following three conceptual models that have been applied to the understanding of indirect self-destructive and life-threatening behavior:

1. *Passive Suicide*: Some of the earliest investigators of ILTB note that an obvious result of much of this behavior is an increased probability and acceleration of death, and therefore have interpreted it to be a form of passive or subintentional suicide (Shniedman, 1968; Farberow, 1982; Farberow & Nehemkis, 1979).

2. *Noncompliance*: A number of researchers have conceptualized these behaviors as a problem of patient noncompliance. Proponents of this explanation are focused on medical noncompliance and have noted several variables that can contribute to the behavior. Parkin, Henney, Quirk, and Crooks (1976) found that chronically ill older adults who failed to take their medications as prescribed (despite understanding their doctor's instructions) were prescribed a greater number of medications than compliant patients. Similarly, a greater number of both doctors and pharmacies predicted intentional non-adherence to doctors' recommendations in another sample of ill elderly patients (Cooper, Love, & Raffone, 1982). An older person may have a harder time understanding and remembering his doctor's instructions due not only to reduced memory capacity and general cognitive decline, but also to problems communicating with the doctor. Difficulties in communication would understandably make it more difficult for a physician to assuage any suspicions or concerns, thus activating personality traits which may contribute to noncompliance, such as suspiciousness and paranoia.

3. *Personal Control*: Extensive analysis of the phenomenon of self-injurious actions indicates a third possible conceptualization of the purpose of this behavior–that older adults often jeopardize their physical well-being in an attempt to gain control over what they perceive to be a negative life situation (Kastenbaum & Mishara, 1971). These investigators have concluded that one purpose of ILTB behavior is to increase attention from staff and thus actually prolong survival. This alternative conceptualization is particularly helpful for understanding cases of ILTB in which there is no evidence that the patient wishes to die. In these cases ILTB may actually represent an attempt by the

patient to control or change her circumstances or to communicate his needs to people who have control over them. Thibault (1984) analyzed and developed a treatment modality for patients engaging in ILTB in a family medicine setting, using single-subject design methodology. Results revealed that in all five cases, issues of personal control and problem-solving were central to both the development and the cessation of the behaviors. Each patient was attempting to change an unacceptable life situation by using ILTB.

CASE REPORT

An 86-year-old female, S. G., had enjoyed a lifetime of unusually good mental and physical health, had taken no medications, and had sought no medical attention prior to the day of her hospital admission. Accompanied by her sister-in-law, she had presented herself earlier in the day at a private physician's office complaining of weakness, which had progressed over the past four weeks. During this time the patient had fallen to the floor occasionally while ambulating and in the past twenty-four hours she had suffered two falls. Her sister-in-law noted that S. G. had recently shown brief signs of confusion, which were episodic but increasing in number along with her weakness. The patient had no significant past medical history other than partial deafness in one ear, which was caused by an accident in childhood but had been adequately compensated by a hearing aid. The patient had never married and presently resided independently in a continuing care retirement community, her home for the past nine years.

The physical examination revealed a well-developed, well-nourished female in no acute distress, who was moderately mentally confused and preoccupied with her hearing aid. She was afebrile; blood pressure was 125/75 mm Hg with no postural change; pulse was 130 beats per minute and respirations were 20 per minute and regular. The physical examination was otherwise unremarkable. Routine blood tests, chest x-ray, electrocardiogram, and echocardiogram were performed. The admitting physician's impression of her diagnosis was dementia, tachycardia of unknown etiology, and atherosclerotic cardiovascular disease (ASCD).

On the night of admission the patient was placed on Lanoxin and was evaluated by a cardiologist the following day. A diagnosis of supraventricular tachycardia was made. Lanoxin was increased and

Procan SR was added to the treatment regimen. A routine urinalysis revealed pyuria with the urine growing Escherichia coli. The patient was treated with an oral antibiotic. During the course of her hospital stay the patient was also evaluated for occult blood in the stool with an upper and lower GI series and sigmoidoscopy. The upper GI was "consistent with inflammation and perhaps small ulceration in the area of upper duodenum." Riopan was prescribed for the patient. Benadryl and Asendin were added to the treatment regimen for undocumented reasons. After a four-day hospital stay the patient's mental confusion improved but her physical weakness persisted. She was transferred to the nursing home section of her retirement community because her physician believed that the patient would probably never walk alone. The final note in her chart stated that he expected the patient "to have a progressive downhill course." This physician did not continue her care. Upon discharge from the hospital S. G. became a patient of the medical director of the nursing facility.

In the nursing home the patient was initially described as cooperative and ambulatory; however, her behavior began to deteriorate, resulting in combative episodes involving nursing personnel. Haldol was given for sedation. Seven weeks after her discharge from the hospital the patient refused to go to meals. Bedside feeding using an Asepto syringe was initiated. The patient was uncooperative, spat the food, required restraints and increased sedation, and grew weaker. During a forced feeding in the eighth week after discharge from the hospital the patient aspirated and died. Medical autopsy revealed the cause of death to be food aspiration.

On the day prior to her death the family had requested that a university-based geriatrician offer a second opinion of S. G.'s condition. He had just one opportunity to assess the patient and had asked the clinical gerontologist to assess her mental status on a STAT basis. The patient died just hours before this could be accomplished.

Subsequently, the clinical gerontologist conducted a social autopsy. Information was gleaned from the nursing home chart with additional material obtained from interviews with staff and the patient's sister-in-law. This analysis of the events leading to death revealed that S. G. had been a very independent, highly intelligent woman who, after earning an M.A. in political science, taught at a major university for forty years. In addition, she had been very active in the Civil Rights Movement during the 1960s. Until her hospitalization she had been an active member of the League of Women Voters, a participant on three voluntary boards, and a discussion group leader for her church. Four weeks prior to medical treatment, S. G. tripped and fell over a chair while attempting to go to the toilet at night. She experienced subsequent weakness and fell three additional times; yet, she continued to function independently in all of the basic and instrumental activities of daily living until the day of her office visit.

Although her mental status while in the hospital was characterized by confusion, this improved before discharge. Assessment of mental status change was made by observation alone. No mental status screening instrument was used. S. G. was presumed to have dementia on the basis of age, a relatively cursory medical history, and normal neurological examination. The physician, who had not known her prior to her illness, failed to consider a diagnosis of delirium and pursue a potentially correctable etiology. In addition, he had not asked about her prior level of activity or education, nor had this information been provided by any of the family members.

On the basis of this diagnosis and because of her weakness, S. G.'s physician advised her family to discharge her to the nursing facility of her life-care community. Acting on this information, S. G.'s family gave up her apartment and dispersed her furniture among various nieces and nephews. S. G. was told that she would remain in the nursing facility only until she regained her strength. She accepted this decision without complaint.

After one week in the nursing home, S. G.'s mental and physical status continued to improve; she was ambulatory with a cane and independently performed all activities of daily living with the exception of tub bathing. This improvement in condition coincided with the resolution of her urinary tract infection.

The social service evaluation described her at that time as being "very alert, oriented in all three spheres, logical, independent, friendly, cooperative and a very confident individual." The only negative comment was that S. G. "feels this is an inadequate environment to meet her needs" and that "she has plans to return to her apartment on this campus." Nursing, dietary, activity, and physical therapy staff wrote similar reports.

During the fourth week of her nursing home placement, after many demands to return to her apartment, her sister-in-law informed S. G. of the permanency of her situation. She became very angry and demanded that the family find her a new apartment and refurnish it in the same way as her old apartment. When they refused, she consulted her physician, the director of nurses, and her attorney–all to no avail. At this point she told a visiting friend that if her wishes were not taken seriously, she would force the issue by refusing all food. She had a prior history of fasting for political purposes as part of her Civil Rights activities. S. G. acted upon her threat and readily explained the reason for her life-threatening behavior to family, friends, and staff. At no time were those discussions documented in the chart.

As time passed and her wishes were neither respected nor taken seriously, S. G. became increasingly hostile and her self-destructive behavior escalated. She initially refused to eat, then to drink. Next, she disengaged in all activities including physical therapy. She lashed out verbally, spit out fluids urged on her and pushed away staff trying to coax her to feed and ambulate. Haldol was increased. She became increasingly weak and Asepto forced feedings were ordered. Four weeks after being informed she would not be allowed to return to an independent living situation, S. G. died while being force fed.

DISCUSSION

A question that arises from the investigation of ILTB is: Why do some aged patients resort to the use of dangerous behaviors and abandon acceptable problem-solving techniques? In their development of a general framework for self-neglect Rathbone-McCuan and Bricker-Jenkins (1992) state that if people are no longer able to protect themselves from age-related crises and losses, they will find new ways to take care of themselves, even if these do not appear "normal" to others. Compared to the active, healthy, young adult, older persons have a diminished repertoire of problem solving options as a result of losing physical strength, income, and other sources of personal power. The individual confined to the hospital or nursing home has even further limitations placed on her problem-solving options. Health care providers often communicate with the family of an aged patient about disposition and management, yet fail to involve the patient in the decision-making process. The person's personal wishes, preferences, and values may never be assessed and considered when attempting to match her need for care with available resources.

When decisions are made without the input of the person, major problems arise in the person-to-environment fit. The patient's first attempt to solve a problem that emerges is usually reasonable self-assertion, expressed to family, friends, staff, or physician. If this fails to produce the desired change, assertion escalates to complaint. Normally, little tolerance is extended to the complainer by the institutional staff. Medical personnel tend to ignore complaints and justify ignoring them by labeling the patient as "confused" or "crotchety." Such labels nullify the person's future complaints. If the patient has no advocate who will take the time to listen and to act on the problem; if she does not have the strength or the freedom to physically remove herself from an undesirable living situation; if because of ageism she is viewed as inferior, weak, and incompetent, she is essentially disenfranchised. If she does not have enough money to exercise other options, then the patient is in a helpless and hopeless condition. The balance of power is not equal between patient and institution.

The entire institutional milieu speaks to the fact that the person is no longer in charge of environment, nourishment, social activity, and even physical well-being. The only remaining power she retains is in the control she exerts over her own body–her intake and output.

The patient is now forced to revert to developmentally primitive behavior to communicate the importance of her wishes. Sometimes this protest is expressed externally and interpreted as aggressive or combative behavior–e.g., striking out, disobeying rules, and defecation in inappropriate locations. More often, behavior is directed against the self. Relying on the belief that her caretakers do not want her to die, often not realizing that she is in real danger of death, the patient exerts control over the continuation of her very existence (Thibault, 1984). She may refuse to eat or to take medications. At this point the patient is thought to be engaging in passive suicide or intractable noncompliance, and the frustration for health care personnel is enormous. Attention is deflected even further from the cause of the problem by attendance to such related legal issues as client self-determination to end life and the question of mental incompetence.

Such indirect behaviors do not cause immediate death but may result in death through the erosion of health over a variable length of time. Indirect life-threatening behavior often stems from a complex attempt to change a negative life situation, rather than simple noncompliance with an unwanted therapy or even the desire to end life, such as in passive suicide. It is only when behaviors become overtly self-destructive or obnoxious to others that the patient is taken seriously.

Sometimes the person's complaint is heard, respected, and acted upon. All too often the response comes in the form of condescending care, tranquilizing medications, and force-feeding.

CONCLUSION

When confronted with a person who is engaging in an indirect life-threatening activity, the health care provider's analysis is crucial to discovering the purpose of the behavior. The physician is of great symbolic importance to the elderly patient and often represents a parental figure (which in itself can be a source of the problem). In many cases–especially when the patient has outlived family and friends–the physician or nurse is the only person who knows the patient well. The elderly person may seek the medical attention and support by engaging in negative health behaviors when positive ones have had no effect. Therefore, the clinician who is treating such elderly patients must take the time to be knowledgeable about and sensitive to the quality of her/his life situation. Merely asking the question, "Can you tell me why you are doing these things that could eventually cause your death?" may elicit the cause of the behavior. Often the services of a psychologist or social worker may be helpful when the etiology of the behavior is not readily ascertained. If the cause of ILTB is not addressed, the life-threatening behavior may continue and ultimately result in repeated hospitalizations, severe impairment of the patient/provider relationship, or, as in the case of our patient, death.

REFERENCES

Cooper, J., Love, D., & Raffone, P. (1982). Intentional prescription nonadherence (noncompliance) by the elderly. *Journal of the American Geriatrics Society, 30*, 329-333.

Farberow, N. (1982). *The many faces of suicide: A study of indirect life-threatening behavior.* New York: McGraw-Hill.

Farberow, N., Mackinnon, D., & Nelson, F. (1977). Suicide: Who's counting? *Public Health Reports, 92*, 223-232.

Farberow, N., & Moriwaski, S. (1975). Self-destructive crises in the older person. *The Gerontologist, 15*, 333-337.

Farberow, N., & Nehemkis, A. (1979). Indirect self-destructive behavior in patients with Buerger's disease. *Journal of Personality Assessment, 43*, 86-96.

Farberow, N., Stein, K., Darbonne, A., & Hirsch, S. (1970). Indirect self-destructive behavior in diabetic patients. *Hospital Medicine, 6,* 123-133.

Gerber, K., Nehemkis, A., Farberow, H., & Williams, J. (1981). Indirect self-destructive behavior in chronic hemodialysis patients. *Suicide and Life-Threatening Behavior, 11,* 31-42.

Gruman, C.A., Stern, A.S., & Caro, F.G. (1997). Self-neglect among the elderly. A distinct phenomenon. *Journal of Mental Health and Aging, 3,* 309-323.

Kastenbaum R., & Mishara B. (1971). Premature death and self-injuries behavior in old age. *Geriatrics, 26,* 71-81.

Longress, J. (1994). Self-neglect and social control: A modest test of an issue. *Journal of Gerontological Social Work, 22,* 3-20.

MacMillan, D., & Shaw, P. (1996). Senile breakdown in standards of personal and environmental cleanliness. *British Medical Journal, 2,* 227-229.

Meerloo, J. (1968). Hidden suicide. In H. Resnik (Ed.), *Suicidal behavior: Diagnosis and management.* (pp. 82-89). Boston: Little, Brown & Company.

Menninger, K. (1938). *Man against himself.* New York: Harcourt, Brace & World.

Mishara, B., & Kastenbaum, R. (1973). Self-injurious behavior and environmental changes in the institutionalized elderly. *Aging and Human Development, 4,* 133-145.

Nelson, F., & Farberow, N. (1980). Indirect self-destructive behavior in the elderly nursing home patient. *Journal of Gerontology, 35,* 949-957.

Nelson, F., & Farberow, N. (1997). Indirect suicide in the elderly chronically ill patient. In K. A. Achte & J. Lonnqvist (Eds.), *Suicide research,* (pp. 125-139). Helsinki: Psychiatria Fennica.

Parkin, D., Henney, D., Quirk, J., & Crooks, J. (1976). Deviation from prescribed drug treatment after discharge from hospital. *British Medical Journal, 2,* 686-688.

Rathbone-McCuan, E., & Bricker-Jenkins, M. (1992). A general framework for elder self-neglect. In E. Rathbone-McCuan, R. Fabian (Eds.), *Self-Neglecting Elders* (pp. 13-24). New York: Auburn House.

Reed, P., & Leonard, V. (1989). An analysis of the concept of self-neglect. *Advanced Nursing Science, 12,* 39-53.

Shneidman, E. (1968). Orientations toward death: A vital aspect of the study of lives. In H. Resnick (Ed.), *Suicidal behaviors: Diagnosis and management.* Boston: Little, Brown & Company.

Thibault, J. (1984). The analysis and treatment of indirect self-destructive behaviors in the elderly Unpublished doctoral dissertation, University of Chicago, Chicago, IL.

Ethics and Aging: Confronting Abuse and Self-Neglect

Paul D. Simmons, PhD
James G. O'Brien, MD

SUMMARY. Self-neglect inevitably poses ethical dilemmas for those involved in providing help. The balance between respect for the autonomy of the victim and the desire to act in a beneficent manner oftentimes results in disagreement and tension. The issue of refusal of treatment and the determination of decisional capacity are explored. Advocacy for the victim in the least intrusive manner is recommended. *[Article copies available for a fee from The Haworth Document Delivery Service: 1-800-342-9678. E-mail address: getinfo@haworthpressinc.com <Website: http://www.haworthpressinc.com>]*

KEYWORDS. Self-neglect, ethics, beneficence, patient autonomy

INTRODUCTION

Few cases cause the sharp pains of internal conflict and emotional distress for professional health care personnel than those involving patients who are deteriorating as a result of self-neglect. They come to the attention of hospitals or social agencies because a health problem has forced them to seek attention. But they are not always entirely willing or cooperative patients. Such persons may have a strong sense of self and profound feelings of what they will or will not tolerate. The very fact they have lived independently and fared reasonably well for many years inclines some older persons to think they can continue to do so without paternalistic care or medical interventions.

The health care professional confronts a variety of scenarios each with its own distinctive factors, but all with certain factors in common. Elements of self-determination, personal independence, personal eccentricities and lifestyle choices, and conditions needing medical attention come together. To these must be added the laws and regulations of state statutes pertaining to the protection of adults. The complexities can become so profound and the trade-offs so painful as to create a dilemma requiring the proverbial wisdom of Solomon. The beneficence to which health professionals are committed seems to require intervention for the sake of the health and well-being of the patient; but respect for patient preferences and the rights that belong to personal autonomy may and often do conflict profoundly with medical opinion.

The purpose of this article is to explore certain ethical issues that emerge from an analysis of patients engaged in self-neglect. Ethical concerns are embedded in or arise from the personal dynamics, medical factors, and conflicting values in particular cases. As Jonsen, Siegler, and Winslade put it, "The ethical aspects are seen in the medical benefits, the preferences of the patient, the quality of the patient's life, and the relation between care of the patient and the familial, social, economic, and legal circumstances surrounding the case" (1992, p. 1). No case is simply one-dimensional and thus presents multiple points to be considered in attempting to resolve or respond ethically to the health care needs of self-neglecting patients. Some of the patterns and quandaries presented can be seen in the following case.

THE CASE: AN OLDER PERSON'S SELF-NEGLECT

A 77-year-old male was seen on a home visit at the request of his wife who was concerned about a bleeding ulcer on his chest. He had refused to go to the hospital or see any other physician. He and his wife had moved to a senior center 4 1/2 years previously from Florida.

Since that time he had been in bed other than to use the toilet. His diet consisted of cereal and a banana three times a day. He allowed no visitors and two years previously abruptly terminated telephone conversations with his sons "as it was too much trouble." A neighbor had called Adult Protective Services who conducted an investigation and declared him competent. They were dismissed by Mr. V.

He was a retired automobile worker, in his second marriage (1989) and had two sons from his first marriage, who lived in the area. He was a heavy drinker prior to his prostate cancer, which was treated five years before. He had refused surgery but agreed to radiation. Subsequently he developed frequency of urination that had persisted as a problem. His wife said he had simply given up on life since his prostate treatment and gradually withdrew from friends and family.

The visit to the 2-room apartment revealed a small man in bed with long gray hair below his shoulders. Images of Rip Van Winkle and Howard Hughes in later life came to mind. He had an unkempt beard that extended to his waist and was matted to a hemorrhagic ulcerated cauliflower lesion on his sternum. He had similar lesions on his left ear and forehead. His nails were long and filthy. His general hygiene was poor. The bedclothes were stained with blood and pus, and there was a stench in the room. The room was absent of any type of materials that would stimulate the mind or indicate an interest in life. There was no television, radio, or reading material in his room whereas the rest of the apartment was tidy and well appointed.

Mr. V. was coherent and oriented. He was able to describe his past medical history in detail. He felt the prostate cancer had destroyed his life. He denied being depressed but admitted there was nothing to which he looked forward. He denied being suicidal. He did not read, listen to the radio, or watch TV. He did not like the bleeding and agreed to be hospitalized and have the tumors removed if necessary. After treatment for the prostate cancer, he had given his wife power of attorney but in a rage later destroyed the document.

He was admitted to the hospital and after two days of cleansing, hair cutting and shaving had three squamous cell tumors removed by plastic surgery. His mental status assessment revealed a high normal score. He refused to see a social worker, psychiatrist, and pleaded with the physician to not notify Adult Protective Services (which is mandated by state law).

He was discharged to return to his apartment but with no medication. Subsequently his wife called and requested that an antidepressant be prescribed which she said she would administer unbeknownst to him by concealing it in his food. The physician refused the request on ethical grounds.

Approximately one year later, the physician was again requested by Mrs. V. to visit, as he had become so weak he was no longer able to get out of the bed. He was now incontinent of urine and stool. He was seen and agreed to be hospitalized. He had atrial fibrillation with a rapid ventricular response. When offered an Advance Directive on admission, he requested that he not be resuscitated and would refuse life-sustaining treatments if they were deemed necessary during hospitalization. Hours later he suffered an embolic stroke that rendered him aphasic. He became more somnolent and was unable to communicate. He was moved to the ICU where he regained his speech but continued to be bed-bound. He was heparinized and a feeding tube was inserted as his oral intake was inadequate and he had difficulty swallowing. He was also started on an antidepressant. He subsequently was transferred to a geropsychiatry unit at his wife's request.

TRUTH, DIGNITY, AND RESPECT FOR THE PERSON

This story poses issues pertaining to lifestyle choices and their relation to human health. It also embodies issues pertaining to human autonomy and personal dignity and the variety of ways in which these may be denied and/or respected. It thus sets a context for considering certain ethical issues related to health care for older adults. Such cases illustrate the ways in which health care providers confront ethical issues in everyday clinical practice. The story teems with matters relating to the respect or due regard owed older persons if they are to be treated truly as persons. As such, definitions of dignity will be important. And some assessment of the importance of the social context in which we institutionalize protections and supports for vulnerable individuals must be made. The aim is to recognize the many dimensions in which we personalize or fail to recognize the demands placed upon us by the respect and care necessary for the ethical treatment of older persons.

THERAPY AND THE ETHICS OF DECEPTION

One issue posed in this case is that of the ethics of truth-telling. Mrs. V. perceived her husband to be depressed and thus wanted him to receive medication for his depression. Since he refused such treatment, she proposed to mix it with his food and thus "administer" it without his knowledge. Her motives were laudable enough and seemed consistent with his own interests. His withdrawal from life was distressing to observe and created additional burdens for her. She was being deprived of his companionship and the personal interactions that create and enhance an environment of mutual enjoyment and happiness. Positive personal relationships contribute to good health in a variety of ways but, at a minimum, increase energy and the will to live and enjoy one another. Mr. V.'s decision to withdraw had a major impact on his spouse. She was undoubtedly seeking relief for herself as well as therapy for her husband.

Even so, providing medications covertly, i.e., without the knowledge or permission of the patient, raises the question of the ethics of truth-telling and honesty. Truth telling deals not only with what might be said, but something that might be done. The temptation is to do whatever works to pursue the goals of therapy. Certainly an effort should be made to overcome patient resistance when health is at stake. But can beneficence justify deception for the sake of caring for a self-neglecting older adult?

Those who support either withholding information or using deception in order to treat, believe that truth is not an absolute requirement. They argue that self-neglecting patients are creating preventable problems for themselves and unnecessary burdens for their family and/or health providers. Issues of justice are also embedded in self-neglect since the cost of care and treatments inevitably increase. For such reasons, using deceptive interventions or manipulating the patient have a strong appeal. Deception is seen as being in the interests of patient well-being or protecting them from self-inflicted harm. Such actions are rooted in the moral commitments of medicine. Thus deception is seen as virtuous, much less justifiable (Meyer, 1968).

Such paternalism seems unwarranted, however, in the case of a patient who is lucid and hardly engaged in behavior that is overtly injurious to self or others. Mr. V. showed a high normal score on his mental status assessment. In addition, he seemed aware of his situation and the consequences of decisions he was making. Deception under such circumstances, warns Sissela Bok (1978), tends to turn into contempt for the patient. If exposed, a deception will also undermine the trust upon which the relation between patient and physician is built. Certainly it makes a mockery of the notion of informed consent by which the patient enters into medical care.

TRUTH AND THE PATIENT AS PERSON

At an even more profound level, the practice of deception is a denial of the patient as person (Ramsey, 1970), which is the foundational issue in medical ethics. The first meaning of autonomy in medical ethics is that the patient is to be treated with respect as a person. Practicing deception assumes the patient is incapable of entering a responsible and mature relationship in which information is freely and openly shared and decisions are reached through dialogue and negotiation. If patients are to share in the decision-making process, they cannot be treated as if they were not capable of handling delicate information or bearing the consequences of personal decisions. What is at stake is nothing else than the recognition of the dignity of the patient.

To be sure, human dignity is used in a variety of ways. Meanings range from the honor or rank accorded a dignitary to a strong sense of self worth. Dignity may also refer to a special endowment from God that confers certain inalienable rights (Congregation for the Doctrine of the Faith, 1988, p. 2; Pope John Paul II, 1995, p. 7). Enlightenment thought stressed the moral worth of the person as a human being. Thus, dignity connotes personal worth and the entitlements, rights, or profoundly personal values basic to the self as person. The four pillars of personal dignity would be: (1) ground-of-meaning beliefs; (2) physical health and bodily control; (3) mental ability and agility including comprehension, integration, and communication; and (4) economic security. Without these, one is deprived of factors basic to meaningful personhood in a social context.

The health professional who uses trickery or deception in the name of beneficence would thus deny the dignity or autonomy of the patient who is acting on his or her own moral commitments and beliefs. Values figure prominently in lifestyle decisions since people act out of their own ground-of-meaning beliefs that shape life commitments.

The patient, after all, may see the issues at stake in much different ways than the health professional who happens to wield considerable power over the (more vulnerable) patient.

If human dignity is protected by openness and honesty, it should also be served by the purposes of medicine. The presumption behind autonomous choice is that the individual is sufficiently free of internal compulsion or external constraint as to make decisions, which are uncoerced and voluntary. Dignity is thus foundational to the ethical principle of autonomy. Without health and strength, one can hardly act as an agent of choice or carry out the actions decided upon. Among the aims of medicine are those of preventing or curing those illnesses or injuries that threaten to deprive one of the factors necessary to exercising autonomy. At one level, the challenge of dealing with older persons is a paradigm of the health care needs of every person, regardless of age. The issue is how medical care might enable persons to preserve personal autonomy.

SELF-NEGLECT AND ECCENTRICITY: LIFESTYLES OF OLDER PERSONS

Lifestyle choices express ground-of-meaning beliefs by which one defines the self and the purposes that give meaning to life. A fine line thus exists between eccentricity and self-neglect. Personal habits that others perceive as self-neglect may be entirely consistent with the pursuit of values important to the person. Gandhi's fasts as part of his social protest movement are a case in point. Even so, self-neglecting behavior has special relevance for the health of older persons. At the extreme, neglect is a form of abuse that results in frailty of body and mind that are not simply the inevitable consequences of aging. One's powers mentally and physically tend to erode as aging advances. But the process can be slowed and sometimes reversed to a degree by healthy lifestyles oriented toward wellness and strength. Both life expectancy and the quality of one's life can be enhanced.

Even the neglect of routine exercise and healthy diet can be regarded as self-neglect. Mr. V.'s medical examination showed no malnutrition; his weakness was from passivity and inactivity. His greatest physical exertion was rising from the bed to go to the toilet or to get something to eat. His meager food intake and routine diet provided sufficient energy and adequate nutrition for what little he did. His wife accommodated his passive approach to life. He seemed to have given up on life and was apparently intent on self-destructive behavior, howbeit through a slow and "passive" process.

Lifestyle choices are thus of concern to ethics. The principle of patient autonomy should include a strong commitment to self-regard (Beauchamp & Childress, 1995).[1] Immanuel Kant emphasized the Categorical Imperative or the absolute sense of moral duty or obligation given to every person (Liddel, 1970; Mackinnon, 1998). An indispensable principle of guidance for that duty, he said, is the maxim that one ought always to treat persons as ends in themselves, never as a means to an end. Regarding persons as ends in themselves is what is otherwise meant by respecting the autonomy, or self-directedness, of the person. Regard for the self is also included in this way of approaching the foundation of ethics and personal dignity. There is, said Kant, a duty to one's own self (Liddel, 1970). The moral principle is that individuals have an obligation to care properly for themselves[2] and show equal regard for the other.

AGING AND THE EROSION OF HEALTH

Caring for the older patient requires special attention because aging is not a benign process. Unhealthy actions or lifestyle choices that are managed reasonably well by younger, more resilient bodies take a special toll on those whose age is more advanced. Growing older brings a predictable erosion of powers that follows no set timeline but is exacerbated by self-neglect. Mr. V. showed the adverse effects of such neglect. Both his cancerous lesions and his outlook on life needed medical attention.

Aging is, therefore, a multi-faceted phenomenon influenced by a number of factors including lifestyle choices, cultural standing, and acute or chronic illnesses. As Dr. Christine Cassel of the University of Chicago put it, "By and large, the changes are decremental. Every organ is losing reserve capacity." The decline toward becoming a casualty is exacerbated by the fact that the aging body does not recover from acute illness as rapidly as it once did. "Aging . . . is first a human fact," says Rosa Herranz. "It is persons, human beings, who age, who feel their own bodies' and minds' growing incapacity and progressive deterioration; who feel, too, their family circle, their economic situation, their work and social structure gradually coming apart around them" (Herranz, 1991).

In Mr. V.'s case, the primary event contributing to his altered lifestyle was prostate cancer and its treatment. His subsequent retreat from life was not from chronic illness or debility but from the psychic and emotional impact of impaired function. He was healthy and strong enough to pursue life in most every way but he had lost a sense of power basic to his sense of self, which apparently caused him to lose most of his interest in life. As in so many cases, many self-abuse or self-neglecting persons are functionally capable.

AGING AS AN ASSAULT ON DIGNITY

Health professionals recognize that aging can be a powerful assault on the pillars of human dignity. The older one is, the more susceptible to disease, dementia, and despair one becomes. When self-neglecting behavior is added to this mix, the problems for the older patient become even more complex.

Knowing the special problems associated with aging helps to shape healthcare concerns. Attention is focused on those areas that make older persons more vulnerable to chronic illness or injury that might severely limit their freedom and mobility. Such care is owed the person because his or her dignity and well-being are at stake. The ethical ground of medicine is that it aims to prevent or cure such assaults against human autonomy. Autonomy as self-governance or self-directedness depends upon one's knowing and being able to do for oneself and others. The ability to know and reflect upon what is known, and one's capacity for gathering, storing, and retrieving information are vital to a sense of well-being. But those capacities are under attack.

Personal autonomy is also defined by the choices people make, since choices express the values by which life is shaped and the commitments that make life worth living. But the capacity for choice is limited to a considerable degree by the ability to carry out those choices. Freedom to act requires that there be no disabling injury and that goals be accessible or that one is not under constraints, either external or internal. Human choices also depend on adequate support from members of the family and those professionals who provide care. Unless one's support system is committed to enhancing personal autonomy, severe setbacks may be experienced that are not always related to bad lifestyle choices. Personal freedoms can be limited from such matters as lack of wheelchair accessibility or the caregiver's use of restraints.

Autonomy is thus related to personal liberties, freedom of movement, association, and the pursuit of cherished interests. The life situation of older patients can be terribly threatening when it is extremely limiting or confining. Dependency on others can be a humiliation that quickly erodes the will to live.

Aging thus contributes to the reasons for which people begin to withdraw from life. Some older people tend to "cocoon" or withdraw to themselves in ever smaller environments where they feel safer and more comfortable. The inability to control one's environment is a major factor forcing people into ever more restricted spaces and activities. In turn, environmental restrictions contribute to the constriction of interests and involvements. The world of the television may become the living environment of the aging who are withdrawing into a world of nostalgia, make-believe, and fantasy. An environment may be chosen that reminds them of a former era in life when they were younger, stronger, quicker, and more energetic; when there were places to go and people to see; when they were less tired all the time; when a purpose for living and going energized their efforts.

ADULT PROTECTIVE SERVICES AND PATIENT ADVOCACY

Restrictive environments may not have been chosen but imposed by controlling caregivers and thus, may be evidence of abuse or self-neglect. For such reasons, many states have implemented efforts to assure that older persons are not being injured or neglected by others in their living situations. Adult Protective Services is built upon the ethical obligation to prevent harm. A number of older persons are subject to abuse and/or neglect and require some agency or person to intervene in such a way as to restore the conditions under which they may pursue a more meaningful and perhaps healthier life.

The statistical picture seems to bear out the validity of the concern. In 1996, 2.2 million cases of elder abuse were estimated, including 1.0 million cases of self-neglect (National Center on Elder Abuse, 1997). These were persons who, though living alone and responsible for their own living conditions, suffered the consequences of being unable or unwilling to provide adequately for their own well-being. Women are victimized by self-neglect more than males, perhaps primarily because women live on average longer lives than men or because women tend to become care providers for a frail spouse or other family member. When it comes to those over 80 years of age, women are two to three times more likely to be self-neglected. The pattern usually involves those who are depressed, confused, or in frail physical condition. Ninety percent of the neglected, however, will come from a perpetrator family.

Being aware of the life situation of the elderly is to grasp something of the dynamics behind the fact that so many states have implemented adult protective statutes. These rules and regulations target domestic violence or abuse and patterns of neglect by guardians or others who have responsibilities for adults (Hyman & Schillinger, 1995). Some states require anyone who has any knowledge of or concern about abuse or neglect to report it to Adult Protective Services. In Kentucky, any person having reasonable cause to suspect an adult has suffered abuse, neglect, or exploitation must report it to the Cabinet for Human Resources. The Cabinet, in turn, must notify police, investigate the complaint, and provide services where necessary, except if the adult refuses them (Hyman & Schillinger, 1995). Physicians are among those required to report.

Ironically, efforts to protect older patients may result in further harm. At one level, the harm stems from a conflict in professional ethics. Among the health professional's ethical commitments are those of confidentiality and respect for patient autonomy. The physician is to be the patient's primary advocate, defending his or her rights to health care and assisting in the pursuit of health and vitality. The conflict is that the state *requires* the physician to act against those standards of medical ethics. Many states have statutes that protect those who report from civil and/or criminal liability as long as they act in good faith (Hyman & Schillinger, 1995), but confidential communications or privileged testimony are not protected. Further, a severe penalty applies for failure to report including fines from $10 to $1000 and a jail sentence or censure that may affect licensure.

The health professional is caught between the coercion of the law and the persuasion of conscience informed by professional and ethical commitments. Not only are confidentiality and patient autonomy denied, reporting also involves deferring to a state agency for decisions and interventions about which the physician or other health care professional may be much more capable. The state's perspective is that the physician is also in a vulnerable situation. The belligerent or recalcitrant patient may intimidate the physician into acceding to patient demands to the extent that the pattern of self-neglect continues. Or, the physician might be reluctant to report an abusive family situation for personal or social reasons, such as embarrassment to a socially prominent family. The Department sees itself as supporting and enforcing interventions that might otherwise be medically and morally mandated and removing some of the burden from reporters who may feel compromised or threatened.

The law undoubtedly has a beneficent intent and may provide positive benefits as health professionals attempt to provide therapeutic interventions. Mandatory reporting can serve a number of goals pertinent to patient well-being. Hyman and Schillinger (1995) mention four: (1) enhancing patient well-being, (2) improving the response of the health-care system to abusive situations, (3) holding perpetrators accountable, and (4) expanded documentation on elder abuse or neglect. However, several conflicts may emerge creating an ethical dilemma. The mandate to report, for instance, may conflict with the physician's judgment as to the best interests of the patient. Or, the conflict may be between the judgment that the patient needs help and the patient's desire to be left alone. Or, the conflict may be between the physician's knowing of an abusive situation and the patient's insistence it not be reported. A physician's decision not to report, while legally problematic, can be motivated by believing that the situation could be aggravated, rather than relieved, by reporting. The situation of the elderly may wind up being far worse off when a report has been mandated. To be required to report tends to belie the role of the physician as the patient's primary healthcare advocate.

The physician who has knowledge of the life situation may be the person ideally positioned to make the most logical recommendation regarding intervention. Some physician discretion seems required by whatever mandate a state might impose. In Mr. V.'s case, it is hardly clear that any benefit would be gained by reporting him to the State. He was cooperative with the attending in every important way, and no other party could be isolated as the one responsible for his neglect. He was his own worst enemy but his patterns of self-abuse were subtle and covert. He was neither self-destructive nor clinically depressed to a degree that affected his ability to exercise independent decision making. An aggressive approach to his care might have alleged that he was suffering from monomania since he saw no great risk to his patterns of withdrawal from family and society. In that case, what might typically be regarded as eccentricity could become an excuse to have the court consider it as a sign of mental illness, take away his right to personal autonomy, place him in an institution, and impose treatments upon him in the name of beneficent medicine.

THE QUESTION OF AUTONOMY: ASSESSING DECISIONAL CAPACITY

The question of patient decisional capacity is also at stake in cases of reporting. The responsibility for evaluating the mental status of self-abusing older patients cannot simply be dismissed as the prerogatives of personal liberties. The consequences of neglect can be far more serious than hygienic and cosmetic problems. Those who live alone are especially liable to neglect themselves, perhaps because they have no one to remind them of their personal needs or to cajole them out of the mental and spiritual lethargy that so easily sets in with moderate depression.

But health care agencies and social services are often faced with persons whose life and health are terribly jeopardized by self-abuse or neglect. Bodily injuries and health care crises dramatically pose the issue of decisional capacity. Cases from Tennessee (*State of Tennessee Department of Human Services v. Mary C. Northern, Supreme Court of Tennessee*, 1978) and Illinois ("The Roby Ridge Standoff," 1997; "Police Rubber Bullets End," 1997) captured public attention when medical and psychiatric problems emerged as a threat both to individuals and the public. Both cases became tragic confrontations necessitated by efforts to intervene for the health and well-being of the individuals. The moral groundings of medicine make it ethically intolerable to be passive in the face of obvious threats to the health and well-being of the patient.

In the Tennessee case (*State of Tennessee Department of Human Services v. Mary C. Northern, Supreme Court of Tennessee*, 1978), Mary C. Northern, aged 72 years, was living alone under unsatisfactory conditions which resulted in her being presented to Nashville General Hospital suffering from a life-threatening infection. Two physicians testified that she had gangrene of both feet probably secondary to frostbite and then thermal burning of the feet. The subsequent infection placed her life in danger. Doctors sought to amputate her feet to avoid further pain and suffering which would most certainly end with a premature and ugly death. She resisted the suggestion fiercely.

Adult Protective Services then went to court arguing that she lacked capacity to appreciate her condition or to consent to surgery. The suit alleged that the amputations were in her best interest and that her refusal should be ignored because she did not understand the severity of her condition or the consequences of refusing amputation. The Guardian *ad litem* responded that Ms. Northern felt strongly that her condition was improving and that she would recover without surgery. She was lucid, showed no evidence of dementia, possessed good memory and recall, was coherent and intelligent. The Court, he said, should find her of sound mind. She did not wish for her feet to be amputated, and her decision should be honored.

The court heard testimony from a physician who found the patient generally lucid and sane. But he concluded that she was psychotic with regard to her gangrenous feet. She believed they were black because of soot or dirt and that the physicians were wrong about the infection. She denied that she would die without amputation. He regarded her as having "monomania" or psychosis in this single area of her thinking. She was thought to be schizoid because she held contradictory thoughts–that she could go on living alone with gangrenous feet and that her future would be relatively stable.

The consensus among physicians was that she did not appreciate the dangers to her health posed by her refusal of amputation. Even so, they acknowledged that she would likely suffer post-operative psychosis and would have to be permanently institutionalized. The court found her incompetent to make a rational decision as to the amputation of her feet and thus ordered the amputation. "She has no wish to die," said the order, "but is unable or unwilling to recognize a condition that will probably result in her death if untreated."

Another case of self-neglect involved a woman in Roby, Illinois. She posed the issue of involuntary commitment for psychiatric care ("The Roby Ridge Standoff," 1997; "Police Rubber Bullets End," 1997). Shirley Ann Allen was a widow who had grown increasingly despondent after the death of her husband from cancer twelve years ago. She lived on a farm outside a small town not far from Springfield.

The trouble started when members of the family heard her talking about helicopters hovering overhead and expressing fears about being followed. On a later attempt to visit her, she threatened to kill her mother and accused them of being impostors wearing masks. The family got together and decided to request an order for involuntary commitment. A judge agreed and ordered her brought to the hospital for evaluation. When her brother and sheriff's deputies went to her home, she met them with a 12-gauge shotgun. A police dog who entered the house was shot. Tear gas was fired into the house and all utilities were cut off in an effort to force her to leave the house. A six-week stand-off followed which became a cause *celebre* by right-wing survivalists who portrayed it as a heavy-handed government action to deprive a person of individual and civil liberties. After "the longest standoff on record" she happened to venture outside and was shot with rubber bullets making it possible for police to take her into custody.

Her brother described the ordeal as "the hardest thing we've ever had to go through." And a step-daughter said, "She's very sick and needs medical attention." Ms. Allen had given ample reason to believe that she was dangerous to herself and others, having threatened to commit suicide and threatened members of the family with a lethal weapon. But even such a necessary and justifiable action is also distressing and disturbing. The patient has been under assault by an insidious process and now she must feel further assaulted by people who care for her under adverse circumstances (Chodoff, 1976).

BENEFICENCE VS. PATIENT AUTONOMY

Overriding the lifestyle choices of a patient can be a serious violation of civil and individual rights, entirely aside from the emotional toll it takes on all those involved. The first principle of medical ethics is regard for patient autonomy, by which the individual's freedom to govern one's own life or self-direction is honored and protected. A great deal of latitude is allowed for eccentric behavior and alternative lifestyles. But that is hardly the end of the matter.

Autonomy and the Right to Refuse Treatment. An autonomous action is sufficiently without external constraint or internal limitations that it may be regarded as freely and personally chosen. Patient autonomy was basic to the "Patient Self-Determination Act" (PSDA) passed by Congress in 1991, which protects the individual's right to refuse treatment in a health care context.

Both the Supreme Court and Congress have affirmed that there are solid moral and legal foundations for protecting the individual's right to refuse treatment. In the case of Nancy Cruzan, a woman who was in persistent vegetative state, the Supreme Court found that she could "refuse" through her parents' decision as long as they could show "beyond a reasonable doubt" that Nancy would not want to be maintained with feeding tubes. It said strongly that "a competent person has a liberty interest under the Due Process Clause in refusing unwanted medical treatment" (*Cruzan v. Director*, 1990). The Court found three grounds for supporting patient autonomy rights in the clinical context: the right to bodily integrity (*Union Pacific Railway Company v. Botsford*, 1891),[3] the right to self-determination (*Schloendorff v. Society of NY Hospital*, 1914),[4] and the right to act upon one's own conscientious beliefs (*Planned Parenthood of SE Pennsylvania v. Casey*, 1992).[5]

Protecting and respecting individual liberties, however, is premised on the ability to demonstrate responsible, that is, non-injurious or non-threatening, behavior both toward the self and others. The physician is often faced with having to evaluate whether a patient lacks such decisional capacity. The process of securing informed consent involves the physician at the point of being certain the consent is genuinely informed and the decision is consistent with value commitments important to the patient. Or, if there are reasons not to abide by the patient's decision, there need to be reasons solid enough to stand up in court. There are serious issues of liability involved in treating patients without their permission to do so.

Self-Neglecting Behavior and Refusal of Treatment. Refusing life saving surgeries might be considered self neglect. Or, it might reflect ground-of-meaning beliefs that should be respected and honored. Older persons might well consider that life has already been lived long and well, and that additional pain and suffering at this stage is hardly worth it. If they have entered the phase of "letting go" they might regard aggressive interventions as unwanted and undesirable. Death might be regarded with considerable equanimity making painful surgeries more to be avoided than the end of life itself.

Even so, it must not be assumed that the older patient will refuse even risky procedures. Their thinking could be some variety of "what do I have to lose?" Or, they might be spry enough still to have a high risk-taking capacity. For the physician to withhold the information about the procedure would be to engage in a form of paternalism. The action would not only be ageist; it also deprives the patient of an exercise in dignity, of affirming his or her own autonomy, that is, commitments to profound beliefs that seem to require or allow the decision made.

A further variable with regard to refusal of treatment is the ability of the patient to articulate decisions in a way that satisfies the expectations of others. Mary Northern was lucid but hardly talkative, much less articulate. Because she did not state her wishes clearly and extensively and because she demonstrated flawed thinking with regard to the gangrene of her feet, she was regarded as having impaired judgment. Her legs were thus amputated. The problem may have been in the level of the expectations held by her interrogators not in the propriety of her decisions.

Had she been clearer about the fact she understood that refusal of amputation meant the inevitability of death, her wishes might have been honored. Decisional capacity is related to the ability to relate actions to consequences or outcomes. A patient with acute myelomonocitic leukemia, named Mrs. D., refused chemotherapy much to the dismay of her attending and the oncologist. Her physician had explained not only that it was confirmed by bone marrow biopsy but also went into detail about the prognosis and interventions available. It was a rather bleak picture. There was a 25% cure rate.

The oncologist made plans to insert a Hickman catheter and begin induction of the chemotherapeutic agent. But Diane refused. She was angry that it was simply assumed she would go for the treatment. She had made up her mind against the chemotherapy. The physician continued conversations with her over a period of days, but she remained firm in her resolve to refuse treatment. The hospitalization would be prolonged and painful. She would lack control over her body. The side-effects of chemotherapy would be unpleasant involving pain and anguish. And, for her, the odds of 25% cure rate were not enough to justify all that she would have to endure. Further, they knew of no closely matched donor for the bone marrow graft she would certainly need (Quill, 1991).

Mrs. D. demonstrated two crucial components of autonomy, agency and action. She did not simply articulate her choice; she was able to act on the basis of her decision. Not everyone is. They may have a disabling physical limitation or a debilitating illness or other severe impairment that simply prevents walking away or acting on the basis of one's choice. Action also means no constraint imposed by one's environment or accessibility to various alternatives one finds more acceptable.

BENEFICENCE, COMPETENCY, PATERNALISM

Respecting a patient's autonomy is not a matter of allowing just anything a patient may decide, request, or demand. Decisions are more a matter of expressing a preference among options than a matter of delivering a mandate (Jonsen, 1998).[6] The fact that patient decisions may be ambiguous and/or physically harmful underscores the need for evaluating decisional capacity.

Such an evaluation is basic to the practice of beneficence, which requires doing good or seeking the well-being or health of the patient (Beauchamp & Childress, 1995). Beneficence may also include nonmaleficence, or doing no harm (*primum non nocere*) and preventing harm where possible (Frankena, 1973). Intervening to keep a person from harming oneself or not injuring someone else is a primary moral obligation as a corollary to doing good. No physician can claim to provide appropriate care for a patient who is allowed to do whatever they want no matter the harm or injury that may happen to themselves or others.

Only a court of law can decide a person's competency, of course. The term is often used but not precisely so in a clinical context. But health care personnel must decide whether the patient's decision reflects a truly informed consent and is appropriate to the information received. A patient's decisions can be accepted as informed, rational, and responsible if three things are present: (1) the ability to understand the diagnosis, alternative treatments available, and their prognoses; (2) the ability to relate personal values, commitments, loyalties, and interests to the medical data given; and (3) the ability to communicate one's decision based upon awareness of alternatives available, personal desires, and their consequences. A patient can refuse even life-saving interventions as long as they demonstrate that they fully understand the consequences–the point at which Mary Northern failed to satisfy her interrogators. The issue is not to get the patient to agree with the physician. An "irrational" choice is not the same as simply rejecting what is regarded as the basic standard of treatment (Brock & Wartman, 1990). The burden of proof is always on those who would override the patient's choice. Even irrational decisions are to be honored as long as they are procedurally sound.

Paternalism enters the picture when a physician overrides patient preferences or imposes treatments the patient has attempted to refuse. Rejecting patient preferences may be entirely justifiable as in cases where threats to the well-being of others or danger to public health are present. Most philosophers agree that personal liberties may be limited by the principle of harm (*Tarasoff v. Regents of the University of California*, 1976). The most benign motives for imposing treatments are those prompted by believing refusal of treatment indicates decisional incapacity or that the illness can apparently be treated and deterioration reversed.

But paternalism may also be prompted by less noble motives. Treatments may be imposed from a "doctor knows best what is good for you" pattern of behavior. Some physicians take offense when patients second-guess or question a recommended treatment. Assuming the authority of specialist knowledge may explain why physicians ignore Advance Directives (SUPPORT, Principle investigators, 1995). A conflict of interest may also be at stake when physicians impose treatments on patients that are of financial benefit to the physician. Or, it may be thought to be in the patient's best interest or that the patient's consent is not even required, which indicates condescension toward the patient.

Again, ethics and the purposes of medicine come together when considering patient autonomy. Ethics insist on the human right of being taken seriously, of having personal choices respected because they are based upon profound moral, religious, or personal commitments around which the person defines oneself. To deny one's right of self-determination is to reject the person as person, to treat them without regard to the dignity to which they are rightly entitled.

A primary goal of medicine is also to restore or enhance the mental and/or physical health of the patient so as to enable autonomous choices and actions consistent with one's cherished values and profound commitments. Medicine is person-centered and its art and skills are to be directed toward the well-being, i.e., the autonomy, of the patient. The ethical practice of medicine requires, first, that patient choices and preferences be respected and, if medically appropriate, obeyed, and second, that patient capacities for autonomous living be restored when they have been impaired or diminished by injury, illness, or other incapacitating circumstances.

CONCLUSIONS

Ethical conflicts among the goals of health care are both predictable and perplexing. Caring for the older patient is an exercise in beneficence or doing good for the patient. Health professionals are morally obliged not only to "do no harm" but also to prevent harm insofar as that is foreseeable or avoidable. The irony is that in preventing one harm, another may be unavoidable. In trying to avoid an untimely or premature death, physicians denied Ms. Northern's autonomy based upon their finding that she had diminished decisional capacities. What is apparently the denial of a basic human right at one level is the affirmation of a basic human need at another.

Whether or not the imposition of medical care upon self-neglecting older patients is consistent with the goals of medicine requires an individual and collective wisdom. We can neither neglect the legitimate needs of such older persons and claim to be ethical nor lightly impose care upon them that they find inconsistent with their own life values and claim to be people of integrity. Such cases will undoubtedly increase rather dramatically as the population of older persons increases and the frustrations multiply over caring for the eccentric or self-neglecting. The task is to take seriously those for whom we care and work out a collaborative and mutually acceptable plan of medical treatment. Where an agreement cannot be reached, the burden of proof must be borne by those who would impose interventions upon them. Medical beneficence must not become a euphemism for depriving older persons of the last vestiges of personal autonomy, the remnants of the dignity by which and for which they have fashioned their lives.

NOTES

1. See Beauchamp & Childress (1995) for the standard statement of the principles approach to medical ethics. They emphasize autonomy, beneficence, non-maleficence, and justice.

2. For a further discussion of this issue, see Cutler, S. & Tisdale, W. (1992). Ethical issues in working with self-neglect. In E. Rathbone-McCuan & R. Fabian (Eds.), *Self-Neglecting elders* (pp. 27-45). New York: Auburn House.

3. "No right is held more sacred, or is more carefully guarded, by the common law, than the right of every individual to the possession and control of his own person, free from all restraint or interference of another, unless by clear and unquestionable authority of law" (*Union Pacific Railway v. Botsford*, 1891).

4. "Every human being of adult years and sound mind has a right to determine what shall be done with his own body . . . " (*Schloendorff v. Society of NY Hospital*, 1914).

5. "The right to define one's own concept of existence, of meaning, of the universe, and of the mystery of human life" (*Planned Parenthood of SE Pennsylvania v. Casey*, 1992).

6. See Jonsen et al. (1992), especially chapter 2, "Preferences of Patients." In the third edition, "patient preferences" were listed before "medical indicators." Shifting the order in which the various components of clinical ethics are considered underscores the point that "decisions" are statements of "preferences," not a clinical mandate.

REFERENCES

Arras, J., & Steinbock, B. (Eds.). (1999). *Ethical issues in modern medicine* (5th ed.). Mountain View, California: Mayfield Publishers.

Beauchamp, T., & Childress, J. (1995). *Principles of biomedical ethics* (4th ed.). New York: Oxford University Press.

Bok, S. (1978). Lies to the sick and dying. In *Lying: Moral choice in public and private life*. (pp. 220-241). New York: Pantheon Books.

Brock, D., & Wartman, S. (1990). When competent patients make irrational choices. *New England Journal of Medicine, 232,* 1595-1599.

Chodoff, P. (1976). The case for involuntary hospitalization of the mentally ill. *American Journal of Psychiatry, 133,* 496-501.

Congregation for the Doctrine of Faith. (1988). *Instruction on respect for human life in its origin and on the dignity of procreation: Replies to certain questions of the day*. Rome: The Vatican.

Cruzan v. Director, No. 88-1503, Supreme Court of the United States, 497 U.S. 261; 110 S. Ct. 2841; 1990 U.S. LEXIS 3301.

Frankena, W. (1973). *Ethics* (2nd ed.) Englewood Cliffs: Prentice-Hall.

Herranz, R. (1991). Bio-medical aspects of aging. In L. Cahill & D. Mieth (Eds.), *Aging* (pp. 3-8). London: SCM Press.

Hyman, D., & Schillinger, B. (1995). Laws mandating reporting of domestic violence: Do they promote patient well-being? *Journal of the American Medical Association, 272,* 1781-1787.

Jonsen, A., Siegler, M., & Winslade, W. (1992). *Clinical ethics* (3rd ed.). New York: McGraw-Hill.

Liddel, B. (1970). *Kant on the foundation of morality: A modern version of the grundlegung, translated with commentary*. Bloomington: Indiana University Press.

Mackinnon, B. (1998). *Ethics: Theory and contemporary issues* (2nd ed.). Belmont, California: Wadsworth.

Meyer, B. (1968). Truth and the physician. In E. Fuller Torrey (Ed.), *Ethical Issues in Medicine*. New York: Little, Brown. (Reprinted in C. Levine (Ed.), (1989). *Taking Sides: Clashing Views on Controversial Bioethical Issues*, 3rd ed. Guilford, CT: Dushkin.

National Center on Elder Abuse. (1997). *Elder abuse in domestic settings*. Elder abuse information series #1. Washington, DC.

Planned Parenthood of SE Pennsylvania v. Casey, No. 91-744, 505 U.S. 833; 112 S. Ct. 2791; 1992 U.S. LEXIS 4751.

Police rubber bullets end Roby Ridge standoff. (1997, Oct. 31). *Courier-Journal*. p. A4.

Pope John Paul II. (1995). *The gospel of life*. New York: Times Press.

Quill, T. (1991). Death and dignity: A case of individualized decision making. *New England Journal of Medicine, 324*, 691-694.

Ramsey, P. (1970). *The patient as person*. New Haven, CT: Yale University Press.

Schloendorff v. Society of NY Hospital, Court of Appeals of New York, 211 N.Y. 125; 105 N.E. 92; 1914 N.Y. LEXIS 1028.

State of Tennessee Department of Human Services v. Mary C. Northern, Supreme Court of Tennessee, 575 S.W.2d 946; 1978 Tenn. LEXIS 693.

SUPPORT, Principle investigators (1995). A controlled trial to improve care for seriously ill hospitalized patients: The study to understand prognoses and preferences for outcomes and risks of treatment (SUPPORT). *Journal of the American Medical Association, 274*, 1591-1598.

Tarasoff v. Regents of the University of California, S.F. No. 23042, Supreme Court of California, 17 Cal. 3d 425; 551 P.2d 334; 1976 Cal. LEXIS 297.

The Roby Ridge standoff is one woman vs. the police. (1997, Oct. 5). *Courier-Journal*. p. A4.

Union Pacific Railway Company v. Botsford, No. 1375, Supreme Court of the United States, 141 U.S. 250; 11 S. Ct. 1000; 1891 U.S. LEXIS 2519.

Alcohol Abuse and Self-Neglect in the Elderly

Richard D. Blondell, MD

SUMMARY. Approximately 1% to 3% of elderly in the United States suffer from the consequences of excessive alcohol consumption. Many more drink amounts of alcohol that place them at risk for alcohol-related problems. Alcoholism is thought to be a significant contributor to the etiology of self-neglect among older adults. Affected individuals can suffer from malnutrition, develop chronic health problems, acquire unintentional injuries, become depressed, neglect their health care needs, and isolate themselves from friends and family. Premature death can result. Professionals who provide services to elderly people with alcohol-related problems have a critical role to play by screening these individuals for an alcohol use disorder and encouraging them to participate in treatment. Identification of and intervention for an alcohol use disorder may contribute to the prevention of self-neglect among older adults. *[Article copies available for a fee from The Haworth Document Delivery Service: 1-800-342-9678. E-mail address: getinfo@haworthpressinc.com <Website: http://www.haworthpressinc.com>]*

KEYWORDS. Alcoholism, alcohol abuse, elderly, geriatrics, self-neglect

INTRODUCTION

Alcohol abuse may be a significant factor causing self-neglect by the elderly; however, this problem may be larger than generally appre-

---

Richard D. Blondell is Professor of Family and Community Medicine, University of Louisville School of Medicine, Louisville, KY 40292.

[Haworth co-indexing entry note]: "Alcohol Abuse and Self-Neglect in the Elderly." Blondell, Richard D. Co-published simultaneously in *Journal of Elder Abuse & Neglect* (The Haworth Maltreatment & Trauma Press, an imprint of The Haworth Press, Inc.) Vol. 11, No. 2, 1999, pp. 55-75; and: *Self-Neglect: Challenges for Helping Professionals* (ed: James G. O'Brien) The Haworth Press, Inc., 1999, pp. 55-75. Single or multiple copies of this article are available for a fee from The Haworth Document Delivery Service [1-800-342-9678, 9:00 a.m. - 5:00 p.m. (EST). E-mail address: getinfo@haworthpressinc.com].

ciated by clinicians and others who provide care for the elderly. Traditionally, research in alcohol abuse has focused on groups of individuals representing the stereotypic picture of alcoholics: the homeless, jail inmates with antisocial personality disorders, unemployed men. Within the last few decades, professionals and the lay public have begun to appreciate that alcoholism casts a much wider net. Many understand that women, successful business people, and professionals are all subject to this devastating problem. Epidemiologic studies suggest that alcohol abuse is more common in the elderly than previously thought. This has led to an increased interest in the identification and treatment of alcohol problems in the elderly and the self-neglect associated with alcohol abuse.

Definitions

Unfortunately, there are no clear definitions of what constitutes "alcohol abuse" or "alcoholism," nor is there agreement among authorities on this issue. These are concepts that depend on the observations of biological, psychological, and social consequences of the repeated self-administration of alcohol. These terms mean different things to the lay public, law enforcement officials, non-medical professionals, and medical professionals. Their meaning tends to vary with the social context in which they are used.

Medical professionals have viewed alcoholism as a disease. The American Psychiatric Association (1994) has defined alcohol dependence and alcohol abuse in the *Diagnostic and Statistical Manual of Mental Disorder, 4th Edition* (DSM-IV). Alcohol abuse is a maladaptive pattern of alcohol consumption that leads to clinically significant biopsychosocial problems. Alcohol dependence is defined as alcohol abuse with evidence of tolerance, withdrawal, and repetitive compulsive use despite negative consequences. A similar disease-oriented approach to defining alcohol abuse and alcohol dependence is taken by the *International Classification of Diseases, 9th Revision* (Public Health Service, 1991). These dichotomous classifications are useful for diagnostic coding for medical record purposes, research, and billing for services. However, they do not necessarily reflect the realities of clinical medicine because there are no categories for excessive drinking per se.

Consumption of alcohol by the elderly can be represented as a continuum. Some consume very little alcohol on rare occasions, others consume great quantities of alcohol regularly, and a number of individuals fall somewhere between these two extremes. The World Health Organization (Saunders, Aasland, Amundsen, & Grant, 1993) defines the "alcohol use disorders" with four levels of alcohol consumption: dependence, abuse, harmful use, and hazardous use. The National Institutes of Health (NIH) (1995) takes a similar approach, classifying individuals as either: (a) "low-risk drinking," (b) "at increased risk for developing alcohol-related problems," (c) "currently experiencing alcohol-related problems," and (d) "maybe alcohol dependent." Although the NIH approach lacks the accuracy needed for clinical research, it does reflect clinical reality. These NIH guidelines consider those aged 65 years or more who drink no more than one drink per day to be low-risk drinkers. At-risk individuals include those who drink in excess of these amounts, drink in risky situations (e.g., before driving), and those with a personal history of an alcohol use disorder who abstain from drinking. This category is similar to the "hazardous use" classification of the World Health Organization. The remaining categories are similar to the DSM-IV criteria for abuse and dependence. One "standard" drink consists of 12 g of ethanol, about 350 ml (12 ounces) of beer, 150 ml (5 ounces) of wine, or 45 ml (1.5 ounces) of distilled spirits.

Prevalence

About 1% to 3% of the elderly are estimated to be alcohol-dependent and 10% to 17% drink amounts that place them at risk for adverse consequences (Reid & Anderson, 1997). These individuals tend to be over-represented in health care settings. As a group, the current cohort of elderly drinks less than younger cohorts.

One group of researchers (Liberto, Ostin, & Ruskin, 1992) reviewed 21 cross-sectional studies conducted between 1960 and 1990 that specifically evaluated the alcohol abuse disorders in those aged 60 years or more. Compared with younger cohorts, the elderly used less alcohol, had a higher proportion of abstinence, and had a lower proportion of heavy drinking. The researchers also concluded that older men drink more than older women. Midanik and Clark (1994) compared the results of the national alcohol surveys that were conducted in 1984 and 1990.

Compared with younger groups, those aged 60 years or more had a lower proportion of current drinkers, had a lower proportion of weekly drinkers, and had a lower proportion of heavy drinkers (those who consumed five or more drinks once per week). They found no change between 1984 and 1990 in these statistics. Another group of researchers (Grant et al., 1984) reported the results of the National Longitudinal Alcohol Epidemiologic Survey. The estimated rate of alcohol abuse and dependency in those aged 65 years or more using DSM-IV criteria was 0.64%. This compares with the rate of 15.94% for the 18- to 29-year-old group, 7.27% for the 30- to 44-year-old group, and 3.47% for the 45- to 64-year-old group. Rates were found to vary by race and gender which, in general, were lower for blacks and women. As compared with younger groups, those aged 60 years or more had the lowest proportion of alcohol dependence symptoms and had the lowest proportion of negative social consequences related to alcohol abuse (Midanik & Clark, 1995).

The reasons why the current cohort of elderly drink less than younger cohorts are not clear. It may be that people drink less as they age or that people who consume large quantities of alcohol are less likely to survive until later life than those who drink in moderation or who abstain from alcohol. It may be that different cohorts have different life-long rates of alcohol consumption. As the current cohort of young people grows older and becomes elderly, they may consume more alcohol than the current cohort of elderly people. Graham (1986) points out that there are no good longitudinal studies that provide accurate information about the natural history of alcohol use disorders. Some recent prevalence studies do not provide data specific to the elderly. For example, the National Health Survey on Drug Abuse conducted in 1996 by the Substance Abuse and Mental Health Services Administration (SAMHSA) groups all adults older than 35 years into one category (SAMHSA, 1997).

Although a small percentage of the elderly have an alcohol use disorder, a significantly larger group of older people may be at risk for alcohol-related problems. A study of 270 community-dwelling elderly, aged 65 years or more, found that 17% consumed more than two drinks per day (Goodwin, Sanchez, Thomas, Hunt, & Garry, 1997).

Elderly patients who consume excessive quantities of alcohol tend to be over-represented in health-care settings. However, evidence suggests that these alcohol abuse disorders may often go unrecognized by the physicians caring for these individuals who are hospitalized (Moore et al., 1989). Adams, Yuan, Barboriak, and Rimm (1993) found that alcohol-related hospitalizations are common among Medicare beneficiaries and were similar to those related to myocardial infarctions. They also found that alcohol-related hospitalization rates varied by over three-fold in different regions of the United States and correlated with the per capita alcohol consumption by state. In a study of 5,065 patients of 88 physicians at 21 locations in southeast Wisconsin, Adams, Barry, and Fleming (1996) found that 15% of men and 12% of women drank in excess of the NIH low-risk drinking guidelines. Of patients who present to hospital emergency departments, the prevalence of alcohol dependency may be as high as 15% (Adams, Magruder-Habib, Trued, & Broome, 1992; Tabisz et al., 1991).

Etiology

The etiology of alcohol abuse disorders is not known, but they appear to depend on genetic and environmental factors. Devor and Cloninger (1989) in their review of the literature related to the genetics of alcoholism concluded that the estimates of heritability from twin studies suggest that up to one third of the variance in alcohol-related traits is under direct genetic control. Alcoholism appears to be a heterogeneous problem of polygenic origin, but at least two types have been identified. One termed "Type 1" or "Milieu Limited" is seen generally in men and women aged 25 years or more. It is characterized by alcohol dependence and guilt associated with alcohol use; these individuals, however, tend to function reasonably well in society. The other type, "Type 2" or "Male Limited," tends to occur in males under the age of 25 years. They typically are antisocial and do not experience guilt or remorse over their drinking habits, but they are less likely to become physically dependent on alcohol than those with "Type 1."

Those who study the cognitive aspects of alcohol use disorder stress the importance of learning in the development and maintenance of drinking behaviors (Wilson, 1987). It is a widely held belief that some patients begin to drink excessively after a stressful life event, but an exact cause-and-effect relationship has been difficult to establish (Pohorecky, 1991). Others have found that alcohol consumption and the standards that govern normal and pathologic levels of drinking vary markedly across cultures (Bennett, Ianca, Grant, & Sartorius, 1993). In the United States, alcohol use has been found to vary among different geographic regions, being higher than average in the Northeast and lower than average in the South (SAMHSA, 1997). Family members and peers may also influence the alcohol consumption patterns of elderly individuals.

Pharmacology

Mood-altering substances exhibit the objective pharmacologic phenomena of behavior reinforcement, tolerance, and physical dependence that can be observed in both human and animal models (Carr, 1993). *Behavior reinforcement* can be produced by alcohol, which creates an artificial state of reward through poorly understood neural mechanisms that can lead the individual to drink compulsively. *Tolerance* is the term used to describe the progressive decrease in the sensitivity to the effects of alcohol with repetitive use. It may motivate the individual to take a larger quantity of alcohol to achieve the same desired effect that was previously achieved with a smaller quantity. *Physical dependence* may develop over time as a physiological adaptive state to frequent drinking, which is revealed as the "alcohol withdrawal syndrome" when alcohol intake decreases or stops. Since the dysphoric symptoms of alcohol withdrawal can be reversed or avoided by drinking, there are strong behavioral incentives to continue to drink.

Alcohol pharmacokinetics, (i.e., absorption, metabolism, and excretion) are not appreciably altered with increasing age (Scott, 1989). However, changes in body composition may influence the effects of alcohol on the elderly. Compared with younger people, the elderly have a larger proportion of body fat. This may explain the finding that older men achieved a 20% higher peak in blood alcohol concentration following intravenous administration of a similar amount of alcohol than did younger men (Vestal et al., 1977).

The relationship between age, alcohol, and cognitive function is poorly understood and controversial. Older, heavy drinkers may develop cognitive impairments that are more significant than those manifested by younger drinkers who consume the same amount of alcohol over the same period of time (Ryan, 1982).

SELF-NEGLECT

Self-neglect, summarized in Table 1, is common among those who consume large quantities of alcohol. Those who are preoccupied with the consumption of alcohol pay less attention to their human needs. Some neglect their health and other biologic needs; become depressed; or withdraw from friends, family, and social activities. Low self-esteem is common. The natural history of certain elderly drinkers may result in the "geriatric squalor syndrome" in which elderly people live in a setting of filth and chaos, rejecting all attempts to change their lifestyles (Kafetz & Cox, 1982).

Neglect of Basic Needs

Many elderly people neglect their basic physiologic need for food and water from time to time, but malnutrition is common among those who drink to excess (Hurt, Higgins, Nelsen, Morse, & Dickson, 1981; Barboriak, Rooney, Leitschuh, & Anderson, 1978). Unlike other drugs, alcohol provides calories and can be used as an energy source for an individual's biological functions. It supplies more calories per gram (7 kcal/g) than carbohydrates or protein (4 kcal/g) and can account for half of the alcoholic's total daily caloric intake. Calories provided by alcohol may displace the calories supplied by more nutri-

TABLE 1. Examples of self-neglect among the elderly who abuse alcohol.

Area of Neglect	Consequences
Basic needs	Geriatric squalor syndrome Malnutrition Poor health care Acute medical problems Chronic disease

Safety needs	Unintentional injuries
	   burns
	   motor vehicle accidents
	   drownings
	   falls
	Suicide
	Victim of violence
	Victim of neglect

Psychosocial needs	Depression
	Dementia (Wernicke-Korsakoff)
	Social isolation
	   loss of independence
	   estrangement from family
	   loss of friends
	Low self-esteem

tious food resulting in deficiencies of protein and folic acid, thiamine, or other vitamins. Secondary malnourishment may also occur through malabsorption due to a gastrointestinal disturbance such as pancreatic insufficiency (Lieber, 1995).

Alcohol inhibits thiamine absorption which increases the likelihood of developing clinically significant thiamine deficiency in alcoholics who have a low intake of dietary thiamine. When given glucose-containing fluids, alcoholics who are thiamine deficient can develop Wernicke's encephalopathy. This condition is characterized by an acute confusional state, nystagmus, and ataxia. Wernicke's encephalopathy merges with a chronic condition, Korsakoff's psychosis, and is often labeled as the Wernicke-Korsakoff syndrome. The features of this condition include anterograde amnesia (the inability to form new memories), retrograde amnesia (the inability to recall established memories), and other defects of cognitive function. Patients with Korsakoff's psychosis are usually awake and alert, but are often disoriented to place and time. Unhesitating confabulation occurs early and is one of the most common features of the syndrome.

Other problems that result from alcohol abuse include sleep deprivation and poor health. Acutely, alcohol is a hypnotic and decreases sleep latency, and elderly individuals may use alcohol as a sedative. However, long-term chronic alcohol intake disrupts normal sleep (Johnson, Burdick, & Smith, 1970; Smith, 1982).

Alcohol affects nearly every organ in the body. Some of these consequences are outlined in Table 2. In an attempt to conceal their alcohol abuse, an elderly individual who develops these problems may not seek medical care. When they do go to physicians, most patients will not readily volunteer the fact that they are consuming large amounts of alcohol. Therefore, physicians may treat the secondary problem and not the underlying primary problem of alcohol abuse.

Neglect of Safety Needs

Every elderly person is exposed to risks that could cause harm, but those who drink to the point of dulling their senses magnify these risks and expose themselves to excessive danger. For those who are chronic drinkers, alcohol may become more of a priority than safety. Alcohol is frequently a factor in unintentional injuries, burns, motor vehicle accidents, drowning, assaults (both as perpetrators and victims), and suicides. One study found a dose-response relationship between the

TABLE 2. Effects of chronic alcohol ingestion.

Organ/Tissue	Consequence
Brain	Atrophy, dementia (Wernicke-Korsakoff type), seizures, psychological disturbances
Pharynx	Cancer (especially among smokers)
Esophagus	Esophagitis, esophageal varices, cancer
Stomach	Gastritis, ulcers, bleeding, cancer
Heart	Cardiomyopathy, arrhythmias, hypertension
Lungs	Increased susceptibility to pneumonia and tuberculosis
Liver	Alcoholic hepatitis, fatty liver, cirrhosis
Pancreas	Acute and chronic pancreatitis, cancer
Spleen	Hypersplenism
Testes	Testicular atrophy, decreased testosterone, impotence, gynecomastia
Bone marrow/blood	Thrombocytopenia, macrocytosis coagulopathy, anemia
Skin	Spider nevi, palmar erythema
Muscle	Myopathy (especially shoulder girdle)
Long nerves	Peripheral neuropathy

usual number of drinks consumed per occasion and the risk of fatal injury; persons who reported drinking nine or more drinks per occasion were three times more likely to die from injuries than those who drank less (Anda, Williamson, & Remington, 1988). The risk of death in a fire is greatest among the very young and the elderly, especially those impaired by alcohol because they lack the capacity to take a "mature independent escape action" (Marshall et al., 1998). According to the National Highway Traffic Safety Administration (NHTSA) drivers between the ages of 16 and 24 account for a disproportionate share of traffic fatalities, but alcohol also impairs the driving skills of the elderly and contributes to fatal motor vehicle accidents (NHTSA, 1994).

Neglect of Psychosocial Needs

Sometimes the use of alcohol by the elderly is encouraged by family, friends, and health care professionals as a way to improve mood and increase socialization. However, the effects of chronic alcohol ingestion are the opposite of those desired outcomes. Alcohol abuse can cause depression. Acutely, the neurochemical changes brought about by a heavy bout of alcohol use, "alcoholic sadness," will clear after two or three weeks of abstinence (Smith, 1998). However, chronic use leads to a spiral of loneliness and dysphoria and can be confused with a primary diagnosis of major depression (Bienenfeld, 1987). Chronic alcohol abuse or dependency can lead to significant memory impairment, which intends to improve with abstinence. Alcohol use may contribute to the functional decline and loss of independence of the elderly leading to social isolation (Reid & Anderson, 1997). Family members may seek to intervene only to be rejected by the patient. Given the choice between drinking and family or friends, the elderly person with an alcohol use disorder may choose drinking. On the other hand, the family may reject the patient when they become frustrated after dealing with their loved one who does not want their help.

SCREENING AND DIAGNOSIS

An alcohol use disorder is often not detected in the elderly who more commonly have multiple medical and psychosocial problems. Changes in behavior, cognition, or physical function can be attributed erroneously to the obvious medical problem, while the underlying primary problem of alcohol abuse or dependence goes unrecognized or is treated with a medication. This drug, taken in the face of excessive alcohol use, may only serve to make the patient's medical condition worse instead of better (Hesse & Savitsky, 1987). Patients presenting with self-neglect, falls, cognitive and affective impairment, and social withdrawal should be screened for alcoholism (Thibault & Maly, 1993).

Two types of alcoholism have been described in the elderly population: early onset type and late onset type (Gambert, 1997). The elderly person with the early onset type often has a family history of alcoholism. There is a higher prevalence of personality disorders and schizophrenia in this type as compared with the late onset type. Patients often present with malnutrition, a history of multiple injuries, and a lowered socio-economic status. In contrast, late onset alcoholics have a family history of alcoholism about half as often as the early onset type. Their early life is generally stable and well-adjusted, and they usually are not the typical "skid row" alcoholics. They are likely to be living with family and have a good positive work history. Depression, loneliness, and social isolation are the most common antecedents in both types of alcoholism in the elderly (Schonfeld & Dupree, 1991).

Screening Tests

There is no shortage of screening tests for clinical use. Selzer (1971) developed the 25-question Michigan Alcohol Screening Test (MAST) nearly three decades ago. Although useful in research settings, it was somewhat cumbersome to use in clinical settings. This led Selzer, Vinokur, and Van Rooijen (1975) to develop a 13-item questionnaire, the Short Michigan Alcohol Screening Test (SMAST). A 24-question, copyrighted version of the MAST designed for use with a geriatric population, the MAST-G, is available from The University of Michigan (Blow, 1991). An international group associated with The World Health Organization developed the Alcohol Use Disorders Identification Test (AUDIT), a ten-item questionnaire that is useful in a multitude of cultures (Babor & Grant, 1989). However, shorter screening tests have been found to be the most useful in clinical settings. The most widely quoted alcohol screening questions are the four in the "CAGE questionnaire," developed by Ewing (1984). Cyr and Wartmen (1988) developed a simple, two-question screening test that has been found to be useful in clinical practice. More recently, a single question has been found to be useful in clinical settings, although this has not been tested specifically in an elderly population (Taj, Devera-Sales, & Vinson, 1998).

Adams et al. (1996) studied the problem of screening for alcohol use disorders in primary care patients. They found that the elderly commonly used alcohol in excess of NIH guidelines. They also found that the CAGE questions alone are insufficient to detect such drinking. Asking questions about quantity and frequency, in addition to the CAGE questions, increases the number of problems identified in clinical settings. A practical approach to this is outlined in Table 3.

Assessment

If on initial screening the patient appears to have an alcohol use disorder of some sort, Kitchens (1994) suggests that it is important to ask a rhetorical question: Does the patient have an alcohol problem? It is also important to determine the severity of the patient's problem. A

TABLE 3. Asking patients about alcohol use.

Appropriate initial questions[a]
1. Have you ever had a drinking problem?
2. When was your last drink?

Quantity and frequency[b]
1. On average, how many days a week do you drink?
2. About how many drinks do you have in a week?
3. How many times in the last six months have you have six or more drinks on one occasion?

Patterns and consequences[c]
C. Have you ever felt you ought to cut down on your drinking?
A. Have people annoyed you by criticizing your drinking?
G. Have you ever felt bad or guilty about your drinking?
E. Have you ever had a drink in the morning to steady your nerves or get rid of a hangover? (eye-opener)

a. From: "The effectiveness of routine screening questions in the detection of alcoholism," by M. G. Cyr and S. A. Wartman, 1988, *Journal of the American Medical Association. 259*, p. 51-54.
b. From: "Screening for problem drinking in older primary care patients.," by W. L. Adams, K. L. Barry, and M. F. Fleming, 1996, *Journal of the American Medical Association 276*, p. 1964-1967.
c. From: "Detecting alcoholism: The CAGE questionnaire," by J. A. Ewing, 1984, *Journal of the American Medical Association. 252*, p. 1905-1907.

medical history should be obtained to determine current medical problems and past health problems. The clinician should also determine the patient's level of functioning at home, in his/her interpersonal relationships, and during social activities.

A physical examination can identify the signs of alcohol abuse as indicated in Table 2. Of particular importance is the mental status examination since cognitive defects are common among those who abuse alcohol. Although excessive use of alcohol may cause cerebral atrophy and dementia, patients with Korsakoff's psychosis may not have the general loss of intellectual abilities usually seen with dementia. These individuals do not have a clouded consciousness (delirium), but typically have short-term memory impairment and some long-term memory loss. Serial examinations may reveal improvement in some individuals when they abstain from alcohol, but most do not return to their previous level of function.

Although laboratory values are of limited help in the diagnosis of an alcohol use disorder, an elevated mean corpuscular volume (MCV), elevated liver enzymes, or elevated pancreatic enzymes (amylase, lipase) could indicate heavy use of alcohol. Formal mental status testing and tests of cognitive function to determine the extent of alcohol-related dementia may also be helpful.

Following a medical and psychosocial assessment, patients can generally be grouped into one of the following groups: low risk use, hazardous use, harmful use, abuse, or dependency. The elderly who drink alcohol and who are "low risk" do not exceed the recommended limits for alcohol use, do not drink in risky situations (e.g., before driving), and are free of any adverse biopsychosocial effects of alcohol use. Individuals whose alcohol use can be categorized as "hazardous use" exceed the safe limits and/or drink in risky situations. However, they have not experienced the negative biopsychosocial consequences of excessive consumption of alcohol. Those patients whose alcohol use is classified as "harmful use" have adverse biopsychosocial consequences related to alcohol consumption. Patients who can be labeled as having "alcohol abuse" have a maladaptive pattern of alcohol consumption characterized by recurrent use causing biopsychosocial problems. Patients who are felt to have "alcohol dependence" may have a preoccupation with the consumption of alcohol and a compulsion to drink. They typically show a loss of control over the initiation of drinking or the cessation of drinking once drinking has started. They may exhibit increased tolerance to the effects of alcohol; it takes a larger number of drinks to achieve a desired effect or functioning is preserved at blood alcohol levels that would impair function in a non-tolerant patient. Finally, these patients may show evidence of an alcohol withdrawal syndrome when alcohol is stopped or decreased markedly (NIH, 1995).

Before providing specific feedback to a patient, it may be helpful to classify patients according to the "stage of change" as described by Prochaska, DiClemente, and Norcross (1992). This six-stage model of change (precontemplation, contemplation, determination, action, maintenance, and relapse) has been found to be useful by those who work with patients who have alcohol use disorders. Individuals in the "precontemplation phase" do not realize they have an alcohol use problem and have not thought about changing their behavior. Individuals who are in the "contemplation" stage have thought that they may have an alcohol use problem but are ambiguous about the need to make a change. Individuals who are in the "determination" phase recognize that they have a problem and have made a decision to change their behavior, although they have not taken any action to do so. Individuals in the "action" stage have made attempts to change their drinking behavior. Individuals in the "maintenance" stage have made a change in their behavior and are attempting to continue that changed behavior. Individuals who are in the "relapse" phase have completed the previous five steps but have relapsed to their former drinking behavior. Clinical advice varies with the patient's willingness to change. For example, it may be frustrating trying to convince a man in the precontemplation stage to make a change in his drinking pattern. It would be better to advise this individual to consider the possibility of making a change. However, a woman who is in the determination stage and is ready to make a change might respond to specific advice about changing her behavior or agree to enter a treatment program.

TREATMENT

Brief interventions with problem drinkers are effective in clinical settings (Samet, Rollick, & Barnes, 1996). Motivational interviewing, a directive, patient-centered counseling style for enhancing motivation for change, can make brief interventions more effective by incorporating the patient's readiness to address alcohol use. Even brief advice might have a significant impact on the patient's course of illness. If every physician gave a brief advice statement to every problem drinker seen, the lives of patients and their families would be significantly improved (Fleming, 1993).

Brief Interventions

There is good evidence to suggest that brief interventions work in routine clinical practice in changing the drinking habits of older adults (Fleming, Manwell, Barry, Adams, & Stauffacher, 1999). Bien, Miller, and Tonigan (1993) reviewed 32 controlled studies in 14 countries enrolling over 6000 drinkers. They found encouraging evidence that the course of harmful alcohol use can be effectively altered by well-designed intervention strategies that are feasible in brief-contact contexts such as primary care settings. The practical strategies on how to perform brief intervention have been defined by the NIH (1995) and are shown in Figure 1. Individuals with advanced disease should be referred to an alcohol treatment facility, especially when the risk of severe alcohol withdrawal is significant or when the adverse biopsychosocial effects are great.

Structured Interventions

Sometimes patients with an advanced alcohol use disorder ignore the advice of a brief intervention and refuse help. The families of these people can be referred to a treatment center that will help orchestrate a structured intervention originally developed by the Johnson Institute (Johnson, 1980). It involves convening a number of the patient's friends and family members to meet and rehearse their parts for the structured intervention. Subsequently they all meet with the patient and read aloud letters that explain their caring and concerns. They then voice ultimata, such as "If you don't get treatment I will leave you," (or ". . . will have no contact with you," or ". . . will make you leave the house").

Treatment

Elderly people are often placed in treatment programs along with younger people and treated in a similar manner. However, the elderly have special needs and special treatment programs have been developed to address these needs. Whether these programs will produce better outcomes than traditional approaches is unknown. Participation in self-help groups such as Alcoholics Anonymous (AA) has been beneficial to many older adults, but the effectiveness of AA has not been subject to scientific scrutiny.

Detoxification

Sometimes, an individual will have a high degree of alcohol dependency with multiple associated medical problems and will require detoxification from alcohol in a hospital setting. Thiamine must be given to prevent the Wernicke-Korsakoff syndrome. However, for individuals with mild to moderate symptoms of alcohol withdrawal, outpatient medical detoxification has been found to be effective, safe,

FIGURE 1. A clinical approach for elderly patients with alcohol-related problems. From *The Physicians' Guide to Helping Patients with Alcohol Problems*, by the National institutes of Health, 1995, (NIH publication No. 95, 37-69), Bethesda, MD: National Institute on Alcohol Abuse and Alcoholism.

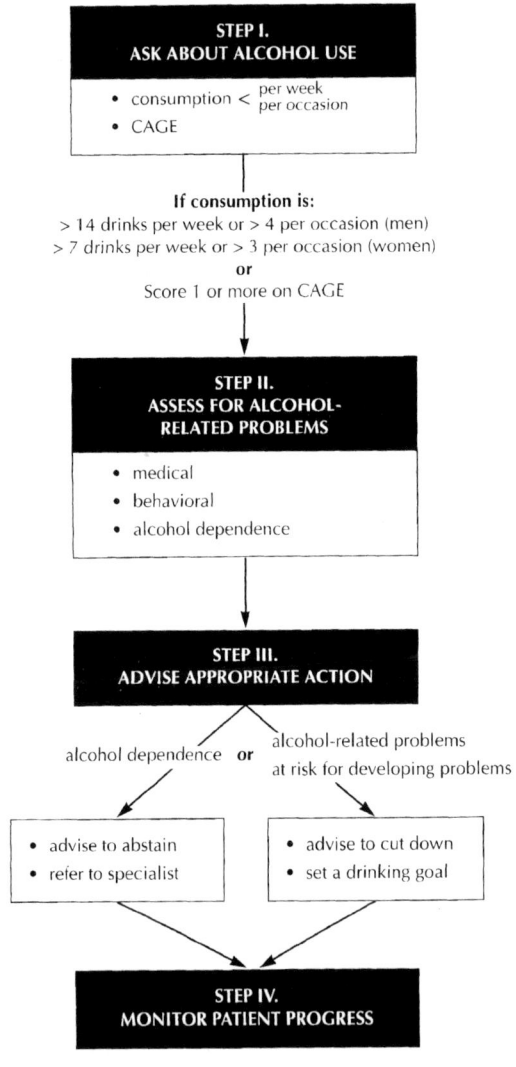

and a low-cost alternative to hospital detoxification (Hayashida et al., 1989).

Follow-Up from Alcohol Abuse

Although there is no pharmacologic cure for alcoholism, naltrexone, buspirone, and acampropsate have proven beneficial in preventing relapses (Schuckit, 1996). Disulfiram may be useful in selected patients, but the evidence to support its use in a geriatric population is weak.

Individuals who are recovering from alcohol abuse or dependency do not drink. They attend self-help meetings regularly, take care of their physical health (including not "forgetting" or canceling appointments), get along socially, function well with activities of daily living, and obey the law. If, at the time of a scheduled return visit, the patient reports failing at one of these tasks, a relapse may be imminent. Primary care physicians play an important role in relapse prevention. Friedmann, Saitz, and Samet (1998) point out that generalist physicians already possess many of the skills necessary for relapse prevention. Drawing on the therapeutic relationship and these skills, primary care physicians have an important role in the long-term management of the patient recovering from alcohol abuse or dependency. It is common for individuals to complain of anxiety in the early stages of recovery from alcohol abuse or alcohol dependency. It is important that physicians not prescribe sedatives, particularly the benzodiazepines, since these medications have been associated with complications, such as falls leading to femur fractures (Herings, Stricker, deBoer, Bakker, & Sturmans 1995) and motor vehicle accidents (Hemmelgarn, Suissa, Huang, Boivin, & Pinard, 1997).

CONCLUSION

Alcohol abuse is not well appreciated in the geriatric population; it may result in self-neglect and in significant biopsychosocial problems in some individuals. It is common enough to be considered in any elderly person who exhibits failure to thrive. Brief, office-based interventions have been shown to be effective in the geriatric population. Astute caregivers can make a difference by addressing the problem of alcohol abuse in the elderly.

REFERENCES

Adams, W. L., Barry, K. L., & Fleming, M. F. (1996). Screening for problem drinking in older primary care patients. *Journal of the American Medical Association, 276*, 1964-1967.
Adams, W. L., Magruder-Habib, K., Trued, S., & Broome, H.L. (1992). Alcohol abuse in elderly emergency department patients. *The Journal of the American Geriatrics Society, 40*, 1236-1249.
Adams, W. L., Yuan, Z., Barboriak, J. J., & Rimm, A. A. (1993). Alcohol-related hospitalizations of elderly people. *Journal of the American Medical Association, 270*, 1222-1225.
American Psychiatric Association. (1994). *Diagnostic and statistical manual of mental disorders*, (4th ed.). Washington, DC: Author.
Anda, R. F., Williamson, D. F., & Remington, P. L. (1988). Alcohol and fatal injuries among U.S. adults: Findings from the NHANES epidemiologic follow-up study. *Journal of the American Medical Association, 260*, 2529-2532.
Babor, T. F., & Grant, M. (1989). From clinical research to secondary prevention: International collaboration in the development of the Alcohol Use Disorders Identification Test (AUDIT). *Alcohol Health and Research World, 13*, 371-374.
Barboriak, J. J., Rooney, C. B., Leitschuh, T. H., & Anderson, A. J. (1978). Alcohol and nutrient intake of elderly men. *Journal of American Dietetic Association, 72*, 493-495.
Bennett, L. A., Janca, A., Grant, B. F., & Sartorius, N. (1993). Boundaries between normal and pathological drinking: A cross-cultural comparison. *Alcohol Health and Research World, 17*, 190-195.
Bien, T. H., Miller, W. R., & Tonigan, J. S. (1993). Brief interventions for alcohol problems: A review. *Addiction, 88*, 315-335.
Bienenfeld, D. (1987). Alcoholism in the elderly. *American Family Physician, 36*, 163-169.
Blow, F. (1991). Michigan Alcoholism Screening Test-Geriatric Version (MAST-G). Ann Arbor, MI: The Regents of the University of Michigan.
Carr, L. A. (1993). The pharmacology of mood-altering drugs of abuse. *Primary Care; Clinics in Office Practice, 20*, 19-31.
Cyr, M. G., & Wartman, S. A. (1988). The effectiveness of routine screening questions in the detection of alcoholism. *Journal of the American Medical Association, 259*, 51-54.
Devor, E. J., & Cloninger, C. R. (1989). Genetics of alcoholism. *Annual Revenue of Genetics, 23*, 19-36.
Ewing, J. A. (1984). Detecting alcoholism: The CAGE questionnaire. *Journal of the American Medical Association, 252*, 1905-1907.
Fleming, M. F. (1993). Screening and brief intervention for alcohol disorders [Editorial]. *The Journal of Family Practice, 37*, 231-234.
Fleming, M. F., Manwell, L. B., Barry, K. L., Adams, W. L., & Stauffacher, E. A. (1999). Brief physician advice for alcohol problems in older adults: A randomized community-based trial. *Journal of Family Practice, 248*, 1378-1384.
Friedmann, P. D., Saitz, R., & Samet, J. H. (1998). Management of adults recovering

from alcohol or other drug problems: Relapse prevention in primary care. *Journal of the American Medical Association, 279,* 1227-1231.

Gambert, S. K. (1997). The elderly. In J.H. Lowinson, P. Ruiz, R.B. Millman, & S.G. Langrod, (Eds.). *Substance Abuse: A Comprehensive Textbook (3rd ed)* (pp. 883-855). Baltimore, MD: Williams & Wilkins.

Goodwin, J. S., Sanchez, C. J., Thomas, P., Hunt, C., & Garry, P.A. (1987). Alcohol intake in a healthy elderly population. *American Journal of Public Health, 77,* 173-177.

Graham, K. (1986). Identifying and measuring alcohol abuse among the elderly: Serious problems with existing instrumentation. *Journal of Studies on Alcohol, 47,* 322-326.

Grant, B. F., Harford, T. C., Dawson, D. A., Chou, P., Dufour, M., & Pickering, R. (1994). NIAAA's epidemiologic bulletin no. 35: Prevalence of DSM-IV alcohol abuse and dependence: United States, 1992. *Alcohol Health and Research World, 18,* 243-248.

Hayashida, M., Alterman, A. I., McLellan, A. T., O'Brien, C. P., Purtill, J. J., Volpicelli, J. R., Raphaelson, A. H., & Hall, C. P. (1989). Comparative effectiveness and costs of inpatient and outpatient detoxification of patients with mild-to-moderate alcohol withdrawal syndrome. *New England Journal of Medicine, 320,* 358-365.

Hemmelgarn, B., Suissa, S., Huang, A., Boivin, J. F., & Pinard, G. (1997). Benzodiazepine use and the risk of motor vehicle crash in the elderly. *Journal of the American Medical Association, 278,* 27-31.

Herings, R. M., Stricker, B. H., deBoer, A., Bakker, A., & Sturmans, F. (1995). Benzodiazepines and the risk of falling leading to femur fracture: Dosage more important than elimination half-life. *Archives of Internal Medicine, 155,* 1801-1807.

Hesse, K., & Savitsky, J. (1987). The elderly. In H.N. Barnes, M.D. Aronson, T.C. Delbanco, (Eds). *Alcoholism: A Guide for the Primary Care Physician* (pp. 166-175). New York: Springer-Verlag.

Hurt, R. D., Higgins, J. A., Nelson, R. A., Morse, R. M., & Dickson, E. R. (1981). Nutritional status of a group of alcoholics before and after admission to an alcoholism treatment unit. *American Journal of Clinical Nutrition, 34,* 386-393.

Johnson, L. C., Burdick, J. A., & Smith, J. (1970). Sleep during alcohol intake and withdrawal in the chronic alcoholic. *Archives of General Psychiatry, 22,* 406-418.

Johnson, V. E. (1980). *I'll Quit Tomorrow.* San Francisco, CA: Harper & Rowe.

Kafetz, K., & Cox, M. (1982). Alcohol excess and the senile squalor syndrome. *Journal of the American Geriatrics Society, 30,* 706.

Kitchens, J. M. (1994). Does this patient have an alcohol problem? [Editorial]. *Journal of the American Medical Association, 272,* 1782-1787.

Liberto, J. G., Ostin, D. W., Ruskin, P. E. (1992). Alcoholism in older persons: A review of the literature. *Hospital & Community Psychiatry, 43,* 975-984.

Lieber, C. S. (1995). Medical disorders of alcoholism. *New England Journal of Medicine, 333,* 1058-1065.

Marshall, S. W., Runyan, C. W., Bangdiwala, S. I., Linzer, M. A., Sacks, J. J., &

Butts, J. D. (1998). Fatal residential fires: Who dies and who survives? *Journal of the American Medical Association, 279*, 1633-1637.
Midanik, L. T., & Clark, W. B. (1995). Drinking-related problems in the United States: Description and trends, 1984-1990. *Journal of Studies on Alcohol, 56*, 395-402.
Midanik, L. T., & Clark, W. B. (1994). The demographic distribution of U.S. drinking patterns in 1990: Description and trends from 1984. *American Journal of Public Health, 84*, 1218-1222.
Moore, R. D., Bone, L. R., Geller, G., Mamon, J. A., Stokes, E. J., & Levine, D. M. (1989). Prevalence, detection, and treatment of alcoholism in hospitalized patients. *Journal of the American Medical Association, 261*, 403-407.
National Highway Traffic Safety Administration. (1994). *Traffic Safety Facts 1993: Alcohol.* Washington, D.C.: U.S. Department of Transportation, National Center for Statistic and Analysis.
National Institutes of Health. (1995). *The physicians' guide to helping patients with alcohol problems.* (NIH publication No. 95-3769). Bethesda, MD: National Institute on Alcohol Abuse and Alcoholism.
Pohorecky, L. A. (1991). Stress and alcohol interaction: An update of human research. *Alcoholism, Clinical and Experimental Research, 15*, 438-459.
Prochaska, J. O., DiClemente, C. C., & Norcross, J. C. (1992). In search of how people change: Applications to addictive behaviors. *American Psychologist, 47*, 1102-1114.
Public Health Service. (1991). *International classification of disease, ninth revision. Clinical modification.* Washington DC: Author. (Department of Health and Human Services Publication No. (PHS), 91-1260).
Reid, M. C., & Anderson, P. A. (1997). Geriatric substance use disorders. *Medical Clinics of North America, 81*, 999-1016.
Ryan, C. (1982). Alcoholism and premature aging: A neuropsychological perspective. *Alcoholism, Clinical and Experimental Research, 6*, 22-30.
Samet, J. H., Rollnick, S., & Barnes, H. (1996). Beyond CAGE: A brief clinical approach after detection of substance abuse. *Archives of Internal Medicine, 156*, 2287-2293.
Saunders, J. B., Aasland, O. G., Amundsen, A., & Grant, M. (1993). Alcohol consumption and related problems among primary health care patients: WHO collaborative project on early detection of persons with harmful alcohol consumption. *Addiction, 88*, 349-362.
Schonfeld, L., & Dupree, L. W. (1991). Antecedents of drinking for early- and late-onset elderly alcohol abusers. *Journal of Studies on Alcohol, 52*, 587-592.
Schuckit, M.A. (1996). Recent developments in the pharmacotherapy of alcohol dependence. *Journal of Consulting and Clinical Psychology, 64*, 669-676.
Scott, R. B. (1989). Alcohol effects in the elderly. *Comprehensive Therapy, 15*, 8-12.
Selzer, M. L. (1971). The Michigan Alcoholism Screening Test: The quest for a new diagnostic instrument. *American Journal of Psychiatry, 127*, 1653-1658.
Selzer, M. L., Vinokur, A., Van Rooijen, L. (1975). A self-administered Short Michigan Alcoholism Screening Test (SMAST). *Journal of Studies on Alcohol, 36*, 117-126.

Smith, J. W. (1998). Special problems of the elderly. In A. W. Graham & T. K. Schultz, (Eds.). *Principles of addiction medicine (2nd ed)* (pp. 833-855). Chevy Chase, MD: American Society of Addiction Medicine.

Smith, J. W. (1982). Neurologic disorders in alcoholism. In N. J. Estes, & M. E. Heinemann (Eds.). *Alcoholism: Development, consequences, and interventions* (pp. 144-167). St. Louis, MO: C.V.Mosby.

Substance Abuse and Mental Health Service Administration. (1997). *National household survey on drug abuse: Population estimates 1996.* (DHHS Publication No. SMA, 97-3137) Rockville, MD: Author.

Tabisz, E., Badger, M., Meatherall, R., Jacyk, W. R., Fuchs, D., & Grymonpre, R. (1991). Identification of chemical abuse in the elderly admitted to emergency rooms. *Clinical Gerontologist, 11*(2), 27-38.

Taj, N., Devera-Sales, A., & Vinson, D. C. (1998). Screening for problem drinking: Does a single question work? *Journal of Family Practice, 46,* 328-335.

Thibault, J. M., & Maly, R. C. (1993). Recognition and treatment of substance abuse in the elderly. *Primary Care: Clinics in Office Practice, 20,* 155-165.

Vestal, R. E., McGuire, E. A., Tobin, J. D., Andres, R., Norris, A. H., & Mezey, E. (1977). Aging and ethanol metabolism. *Clinical Pharmacology and Therapeutics, 21,* 343-354.

Wilson, G. T. (1987). Cognitive studies in alcoholism. *Journal of Consulting and Clinical Psychology, 55,* 325-331.

Community Dimensions of Elderly Self-Neglect

Mary Cay Sengstock, PhD, CCS
Jane M. Thibault, PhD
Rochelle Zaranek, MSW

SUMMARY. Much recent literature has focused on the impact of self-neglecting behavior on elders. Little attention, however, has been paid to the impact of this phenomenon on the communities in which self-neglecting elders live. Family members, neighbors, and service professionals can all be adversely affected by the behavior of these patients. This article reflects on the ways in which the community is affected by elder self-neglect and discusses the inherent conflicts between protecting the rights of the individual and the rights of the community. *[Article copies available for a fee from The Haworth Document Delivery Service: 1-800-342-9678. E-mail address: getinfo@haworthpressinc.com <Website: http://www.haworthpressinc.com>]*

KEYWORDS. Self-neglect, community types, individual rights, community rights

INTRODUCTION

Some service providers estimate that the most common type of elder abuse they observe, as well as one of the most intractable, is self-

---

Mary Cay Sengstock is Professor of Sociology, Department of Sociology, Wayne State University, Detroit, MI 48202. Jane M. Thibault is Associate Professor, Division of Geriatrics, Department of Family and Community Medicine, University of Louisville School of Medicine, Louisville, KY 40292. Rochelle Zaranek is Graduate Student in Sociology, Wayne State University, Detroit, MI 48202.

[Haworth co-indexing entry note]: "Community Dimensions of Elderly Self-Neglect." Sengstock, Mary Cay, Jane M. Thibault, and Rochelle Zaranek. Co-published simultaneously in *Journal of Elder Abuse & Neglect* (The Haworth Maltreatment & Trauma Press, an imprint of The Haworth Press, Inc.) Vol. 11, No. 2, 1999, pp. 77-93; and: *Self-Neglect: Challenges for Helping Professionals* (ed: James G. O'Brien) The Haworth Press, Inc., 1999, pp. 77-93. Single or multiple copies of this article are available for a fee from The Haworth Document Delivery Service [1-800-342-9678, 9:00 a.m. - 5:00 p.m. (EST). E-mail address: getinfo@haworthpressinc.com].

© 1999 by The Haworth Press, Inc. All rights reserved.

neglect (Duke, 1991; Longres, 1994). The examples are endless: the patient who fails to take her medicine, the man who visits the senior center looking disheveled and undernourished, the elderly neighbor whose home is in a constant state of disrepair. In many of these instances, the older adult appears to be mentally alert and physically capable of self-care. There appears to be no need for a caregiver or guardian. Yet there seems to be a constant need for some type of assistance: food, better clothing, a cleaner environment, and so on.

Many such cases appear to result from conflicting life styles–the relative, neighbor, or service provider cannot imagine living in such a manner, and assumes that the elder must be unhappy with it as well. However, older persons who neglect themselves are often content with their life style, and resent even well-meaning outsiders who attempt to effectuate changes. If they are mentally competent, they are entitled to choose whatever style of living they please, although questions may be raised concerning their level of competence.

What is scarcely mentioned in the literature, however, is the impact of the life style of self-neglectful elders on the communities in which they live. While vigorously defending the rights of the older adult, little attention has been given to the fact that some self-neglectful behavior may have a profound impact on the elderly person's family, neighbors, and surroundings. The neighborhood recluse, for example, is a potential health hazard, as her garbage-strewn house and yard may attract disease-carrying rats. And countless hours of expensive professional time may be devoted to the medical care of an elderly patient who has no intention of taking his medications.

Personal rights are not exclusive to the elderly. The community members who live with or near an elder also have rights. Upon occasion, an elder's self-neglect may violate these rights of others. In this paper, we will examine some aspects of self-neglect of the elderly, as well as characteristics of the communities in which elders live, and the impacts which the elders' behavior may have in various types of community settings.

Hence the two dimensions which will be examined are the type of self-neglect in which the elder engages, and the type of community with which the elder comes into contact. An elder who refuses to take medication, for example, may have little impact on the single family home residential community in which he lives; it may, however, have substantial impact on the medical setting in which he is treated, and on family members who provide care. An elder's garbage-strewn dwelling may have little impact on rural neighbors; it is more obnoxious in an urban setting, and especially so if she lives in an apartment building. Throughout the discussion, we will provide case examples of the impact of self-neglect on the community and will suggest means for resolving the conflicts where possible.

TYPES OF SELF-NEGLECT

What the elder abuse literature classifies as "self-neglect" is actually a complex set of behaviors. Reed and Leonard (1989), for example, list 20 separate types of self-neglect behaviors, ranging from direct suicide and covert suicide, through various types of self-destructive behavior, to indirect life-threatening and indirect self-destructive behavior (ISDB). Others have used the term, self-injurious behavior (SIB), " . . . that results in organ or tissue damage to the individual" (Pies & Popli, 1995, p. 580).

A major component of self-neglect, from the standpoint of the health care provider, is noncompliance or failure to carry out the requirements of a health care regimen. Non-compliant or self-injurious behavior has been found to exist from 44% of hospitalized patients in one sample (Kastenbaum & Mishara, 1971) to a high of 88% in another study (Nelson & Farberow, 1977).

Implicit in the concept of self-neglect is the assumption of a *capacity for self care* on the part of the individual. One would not, for example, speak of self-neglect in the case of a mentally or physically incapacitated elder who was incapable of understanding his health care needs or following the required regimen. Consequently, we are necessarily speaking about an individual who is mentally alert and physically capable of caring for him/herself. Whether or not the person does so, however, is dependent upon a number of other factors, the major ones being mental competence and intentionality (Reed & Leonard, 1989).

The issue of mental competence has received considerable discussion in the literature and remains highly controversial. Research shows that most self-neglecting elders in the community do not exhibit mental disorders (Radebaugh, Hooper, & Gruenberg, 1987). Numerous authorities have defended the rights of competent elders to refuse intrusions into their life styles, if they so choose, and most state laws specifically state that services cannot be forced upon a competent older person (Clark, Manikar, & Gray, 1975; Thomasma, 1984; Wrigley & Cooney, 1992). Conversely, others contend that many of these elders may *appear* mentally competent, but a thorough examination would detect underlying psychiatric problems, and would argue that interventions were necessary for the elder's health and safety (Orrell, Sahakain, & Bergmann, 1989; Howard & Bergmann, 1993; Ungvari & Hantz, 1991; Macmillan, 1966). Whichever position one takes in the matter, it is widely recognized as a serious dilemma (Roe, 1977; Thomasma, 1984; Longres, 1994).

The issue of intentionality addresses the older person who is indeed mentally and physically competent, who may understand quite well what is required to maintain his/her physical and social environment and carry out medical and health prescriptions; s/he simply does not choose to carry out the plan. In addition to unwillingness to comply, non-compliance may also be related to such factors as the lack of knowledge or skill or inadequate financial resources to carry out the plan (Reed & Leonard, 1989).

An extreme form of self-neglect has been described, perhaps inaccurately, as Diogenes Syndrome. Initially appearing in the literature in 1975 (Clark et al., 1975), the typical case is a person ". . . characterized by extreme self-neglect, domestic squalor, social withdrawal and apathy, with a tendency to hoard rubbish" (Jackson, 1997, p. 113). Others have termed the pattern "Social Breakdown in the Elderly," or "SBE" (Ungvari & Hantz, 1991a, 1991b; Radebaugh et al., 1987).

Although it is typically seen in individuals who live alone (Jackson, 1997), some have observed the pattern in couples, leading to the concept of "Diogenes a deux" (Cole, Gillett, & Fairbairn, 1992). Case descriptions present a picture of mentally competent, if somewhat socially reclusive individuals with adequate financial resources, but whose house or apartment is filthy and ill kempt, often with human excrement lying around, and with rats or other vermin present (Macmillan & Shaw, 1966; Cole et al., 1992).

For the purposes of the present paper we will analyze these 3 major types of self-neglect: self-destructive behavior, non-compliance, and Diogenes Syndrome, and focus primarily on cases in which the elder is mentally competent and physically capable of self-care.

WHY DOES THE COMMUNITY MATTER?

As noted earlier, there has been scant attention to the impact of elderly self-neglect on the communities with which the affected elders come into contact. Indeed, some might even question why the community should receive any consideration. A common position has been that any interference with an elder's personal choice of life style, or attempt ". . . to force conformity with regard to standards of cleanliness is completely unacceptable" (Wrigley & Cooney, 1992, p. 40).

This extreme position is untenable, however. Communities and their members also have rights. Indeed, many of the individuals whose rights are being violated by the actions of self-neglectful elders may themselves be elders whose health and safety are being threatened. Hence the question arises: Under what conditions may the rights of the individual be abrogated? The only reasonable answer is that individual rights can be limited when they interfere with the rights of others.

Numerous instances could be depicted. For example, limits can be placed on an individual's rights when s/he has a communicable disease that endangers the health or even the lives of others. Indeed, some have complained that the normal public health tools employed with communicable diseases have not been used with AIDS, due to a concern for the privacy rights of AIDS patients, to the detriment of the community at large (Burr, 1997).

Similar impacts on the rights of others may be noted with self-neglect. Indeed, the public health aspects of elderly self-neglect have been noted as one of the few acceptable limits on elderly persons' rights of self-determination (Ungvari & Hantz, 1991b). Thus an elder's hoarded items which present a fire hazard to other residents in an apartment building may present a situation in which others' rights are being violated (Wrigley & Cooney, 1992).

It is our contention that the major limits on the self-determination rights of a self-neglectful elder derive from the rights of others with whom they interact. And these rights will vary depending on the community with which they are involved. We turn, therefore, to a description of the types of communities with which older adults interact and will then proceed to analyze the impact which these types of self-neglect may have upon these communities.

TYPES OF COMMUNITIES

In sociological terminology, communities are "groups of people who share a common territory and a sense of identity or belonging and who interact with one another" (Sullivan & Thompson, 1988, p. 376). In earlier, simpler societies, communities were small, cohesive bands, in which everyone knew everyone else, and they shared a common life style and value system. In such societies, "community" was a concept which included a geographic dimension–people lived near each other– but also had social and psychological dimensions–people interacted with and felt a sense of closeness to their neighbors.

As societies have grown in size and complexity, however, the nature and dimensions of community have changed as well. In the urban settings of today, "community" can mean different things to different people. For many, the "sense of identity or belonging" may not be shared with those with whom they share a common territory, raising questions about the reality of the community experience. Many people search for a sense of identity or belonging with persons in quite different areas. Hence people may find a sense of community with persons in their work place or profession, their religion, ethnic background, or other, non-territorial settings (Broom, Selznick, & Broom, 1984; Henslin, 1999). Some have even noted that the Internet takes on the character of a community (Henslin, 1999).

Consequently, while urban dwellers necessarily are still part of a geographic community in their residential areas, they may interact with them very little and share no sense of identity or closeness to them. Conversely, they may also be part of several other "communities" of people who live at some distance, but with whom they interact a great deal and share " . . . a sense of identity or belonging." As a result, modern urban dwellers actually participate in not one but many communities as they go about their daily activities. And their behavior, depending upon its characteristics, may have an impact on any or all of these.

Hence a mentally alert, physically active elderly person is likely to encounter numerous communities. There are 3 major dimensions on which communities may vary: the degree of geographic propinquity, or nearness of members of the community; the amount of social interaction which the members of the community share with each other; and the degree of identity or closeness which they feel for each other.

Emotionally Close Communities

Communities with which an individual interacts a great deal and in which the members feel close to one another are the type of groups to which most people refer when they use the term "community." In earlier eras, neighborhoods often had this characteristic, and some still do. Today, it continues to be found in the family, which ideally shares a sense of personal closeness, regardless of the geographic distance that separates them or how infrequently they see each other. Other examples of identificational communities are ethnic groups, senior centers, religious groups, or other voluntary associations.

Geographic Communities

Geographic communities are those in which an individual resides; this may be a neighborhood of single family homes, an apartment complex, senior citizens' residence, and so on. A resident necessarily has some degree of interaction with this community because of the common living arrangements. However, residents may minimize their interaction as much as possible and may or may not share a sense of identity or belonging with other residents.

The Service Community

There are other communities with which an individual interacts, possibly on a regular basis, but with which s/he has little sense of identity or belonging. In a work-based community, for example, members may interact a great deal with each other, although they do not live near each other, and may not feel much sense of identity or belonging. Work-based communities may also include outsiders, such as customers in a store, patients in a hospital or doctor's office, or clients in a social agency; such persons participate in the "community" of that occupation, even though they may not actually be members of it or identify with it. This type of community could be characterized as "emotionally detached" because of the low degree of personal involvement which the participants typically share. For purposes of this paper, the service community, which provides medical, social, and other services, to elderly clients is an example of such a community.

Of course, some of these communities may overlap–that is, a geographic or work-based community may also be an emotionally close community. In such instances, it would be necessary to consider the implications of both types. We now turn to a discussion of the impact that elderly self-neglect may have upon these different types of communities.

THE DIFFERENTIAL IMPACT OF ELDERLY SELF-NEGLECT ON COMMUNITIES OF DIFFERENT TYPES

How is a community impacted by the ostensibly private behavior of an individual? Because of the complexity of modern communities, the seemingly private behavior of an individual can impact upon a great many communities, rather than only one. Furthermore, self-neglect which may be relatively unnoticed in one community may engender major problems in another.

Self-Neglect and the Emotionally Close Community

It is in the emotionally close community that the impact of an elder's self-neglect is likely to be felt the strongest. Family, close friends, members of an ethnic community are those most likely to become distressed if a beloved relative or friend exhibits any type of destructive behavior. Doctors and other service providers are often unaware of the extent to which family and friends may already have extended themselves for a patient, to no avail.

An example is Mrs. C., a 77 year-old female, living alone in her own home on an almost abandoned street. She was a diabetic, had high blood pressure and chronic renal failure, was non-ambulatory, confined to either her wheelchair or bed, and unable to manage her own activities of daily living (ADLs). While financially able to hire a private caregiver, she insisted this was not necessary. Her home was cluttered with many boxes, pieces of furniture, and piles of clothing, and was heated by a coal-burning furnace located in the dining room, making for a serious fire hazard. Her only living relative was a son who lived in a city about 300 miles away. He had made 5 separate trips in recent years to try to persuade his mother to update her home or relocate to a safer environment. On occasion she would not even let him in the house. He finally gave up and acceded to her request that she be left alone.

If family members live with or near the elder, they may themselves be at risk. Mrs. S., for example, was a 76 year-old female, residing in her own home with her daughter and preschool grandchildren. She had a history of tuberculosis, congestive heart failure, high blood pressure, and was recently diagnosed with lung cancer. She was bedbound, connected to a catheter, and tube fed. Mrs. S. was oriented and able to make decisions but unable to care for herself. Her daughter/caregiver abused alcohol and drugs. The home was unsafe, with the ceiling caving in, shingles falling off, and roaches throughout. The client smoked excessively in her bed and had been known to fall asleep with a cigarette in her mouth. She had little concern with the condition of her home or the threat which her unsafe smoking habits posed to her or her family.

Other types of self-neglect could also be disruptive to a close-knit community, if the members were aware of it. Like Mrs. C.'s son, why spend precious time or money on food, medication, or other assistance if the relative or friend fails to make use of them? It should also be noted, however, that relatives and friends often are unaware of the life styles of their elderly relatives. An elder may hide the fact that s/he is not taking medications, or be very careful to keep relatives and friends from visiting the home, thus keeping secret the cluttered, roach-infected environs in which they live. As has been noted, some of these patients have probably lived in this manner for several years and may be seen as rather eccentric recluses by relatives and friends (Jackson, 1997).

Self-Neglect and the Geographic Community

In geographic communities, self-neglect behavior may go largely unnoticed a great deal of the time–unless it is extreme and becomes highly disruptive to the life styles of others. Even extremely unkempt living conditions are likely to cause little attention, as long as they remain within the elder's home or apartment. Mr. and Mrs. B., in another case, kept the exterior of their home relatively clean and neat, although the interior was abysmal. Hence members of a residential community may not even be aware of elderly self-neglect, even if it is self-destructive or suicidal.

Only if the slovenly conditions extend outside the home or apartment or threaten the health or safety of others would neighbors become aware or concerned. Mrs. H.'s problem is illustrative. She was 74, a diabetic, with a history of depression and high blood pressure; she was *and* is bedbound because of a stroke. She was not self-neglectful, in that she had her son as well as a paid caregiver to assist her. However, her home, which was already in poor condition, with a leaking roof, deteriorating front porch, and paint peeling throughout, was endangered by an abandoned house next door, which threatened to collapse onto Mrs. H.'s house; the abandoned house was infested with rodents and roaches which migrated to other homes nearby.

This type of impact would be even greater, the closer the neighbors lived to each other. Mrs. S., the careless smoker mentioned earlier, lived in a single family home and was a threat primarily to herself and her family. Mrs. L. also smoked heavily, and, to complicate matters, used oxygen for her lung problems. However, she managed an apartment building; and building tenants were legitimately concerned, even frightened, about the impact her smoking would have upon their safety. These appear to be quite reasonable concerns on the part of community members and call for a public health approach to elder self-neglect (Ungvari & Hantz, 1991b; Wrigley & Cooney, 1992).

A more difficult question, however, arises with the issue of aesthetics. Suppose the elder's non-conformity appears to be merely a matter of personal choice. That is, s/he is not dirty or a public health hazard, but chooses to leave items which the neighbors find obnoxious lying around the yard or hanging in the window. To what extent should community preferences intrude into these persons' life style?

Self Neglect and the Service Community

The emotionally detached community, such as a medical or social agency setting, is a special case. In this type of community, as noted earlier, participants rarely have a strong identification with each other. Doctors and other professionals may only share the work setting and little else. Even more so, agency staff have little sense of identity or belonging with patients or clients, and vice versa.

Consequently, client behavior is unlikely to cause much impact on the service community, unless this is an area with which a specific agency must cope. Hence the staff in a medical agency would become very concerned about non-compliance. And home service staff will be greatly affected by the Diogenes Syndrome client. Entering a rat or vermin infested dwelling, or delivering oxygen to a home in which there are smokers, threatens the health and safety of the service worker. It may lead to workers or agencies refusing to provide further services. The extremely self-neglecting elder may actually threaten the ability of other elders to obtain similar services in the future.

Mr. and Mrs. B. are an extreme example of the impact of self-neglect on a service agency. Both were in their 80s and college educated, with more than adequate income. They were classic Diogenes Syndrome clients: The exterior of their home appeared well cared for, but inside, trash and garbage were everywhere. Protective service workers had to hold their noses when they entered. The couple allowed themselves to be taken to the university medical clinic, where the stench from their bodies and clothing was so overwhelming that other patients left the waiting room. Their clothes were encrusted with dirt and food; their long hair was matted; their skin was gray with accumulated dirt; their fingernails were long and curling into the fingers. They were accompanied by 5 flies that continually hovered around them. When the resident entered the examination room to speak to the couple, the smell caused her to vomit on the spot. Mrs. B. was found to be moderately demented and was placed in a nursing home. Mr. B. insisted on returning to his home where he refused to allow the home to be cleaned. Since he was relatively healthy and mentally alert, nothing more could be done.

Community Overlap

Although we have described these communities as being relatively independent, it is also clear that in many instances, different community types overlap. What can be a threat to the emotionally close community of the family can also be a threat to the geographic or service community as well. The case of Mrs. E. is illustrative. Mrs. E. was a 63 year-old female, residing in her own home with her daughter and young grandchildren. She was diabetic and had both legs amputated. She also had emphysema and asthma and was connected to a vent machine, a catheter, and used oxygen 24 hours a day. Mrs. E. was bedbound and dependent on her daughter for all daily living needs. The home was grossly unsanitary and infested with thousands of roaches on her bed linens and clothing. This situation was certainly unsafe not only for Mrs. E. but also for her young grandchildren. In addition, Mrs. E. had home health aides, who frequently found roaches in their medical equipment and clothing when they left. Because the team members visit other clients throughout the day, both the home care professionals and other residents in the community were at risk of becoming infected.

HANDLING COMMUNITY CONCERNS

As we have previously discussed, a common approach to self-neglect has been to declare the elder mentally incompetent and place him or her in a long term care facility, with objections to that approach being equally strong (Baker, 1976; Thomasma, 1984; Orrell et al., 1989). Clearly, if this approach is taken, the concerns of the community are alleviated. However, there may be other approaches which are less intrusive. Experience with home health care agencies can suggest some of these.

Enforcing Public Health Codes

The use of city agencies to enforce public health codes is always an option if the elder's actions are threatening to the community at large. This approach is most effective in cases of Diogenes Syndrome. If an elder's rat or roach infested home is a threat to nearby property or to home health care workers who enter the home, the city can require that measures be taken to destroy the vermin–or indeed, can enter the facility to handle the problem.

Mrs. D. was a 73 year-old female with a long history of diabetes and high blood pressure, extremely obese, with multiple open skin ulcers on her legs and ankles. On a limited income, she lived in an area with numerous abandoned houses, all of which were infested with rats, roaches, flies, and mice. When the nurse would change Mrs. D.'s dressings, roaches were sometimes found inside the bandages. Mrs. D. claimed that her limited income prevented her from having her home exterminated. The unsafe condition of the home was a serious threat not only to Mrs. D.'s health, but also to that of the caregiver and home health care team. Eventually, the state social services agency paid an extermination company to fumigate the home.

Removal of Services

While no health or social service agency is comfortable taking services away from a needy individual, in some instances this is really what the elder prefers, and may be the only option for the safety of members of any community on which the elder's behavior has an impact. The case of Mrs. P. is an example. She was an 93 year-old woman with chronic obstructive pulmonary disease, asthma, anemia, and urinary incontinence. While she was articulate and mentally alert, she abused alcohol and smoked 2 packs of cigarettes a day. She adamantly refused to move to an assisted living site, although her home was in disrepair. Placed on oxygen because of her chronic obstructive pulmonary disease (COPD), she was warned not to smoke but refused to comply. She consistently turned the gauge higher than needed and continued to smoke. This oxygen supply company finally refused to serve her because of her non-compliance with the smoking ban; a second and third company also refused, noting that they would be legally liable if they continued to deliver oxygen into an unsafe environment.

In the case of Mrs. E., discussed earlier, whose home was also infested with roaches, home health aides made several requests that the home be sprayed. When no action was taken, the home care supervisor made a special home visit to explain the seriousness of the matter and to inform the family that if the home was not sprayed and disinfected, the case would have to be discharged immediately. Finally, they agreed to have the home sprayed and cleaned.

Eviction

In some instances conflict between the rights of the individual and those of the community are such that only a termination of the relationship will solve the matter. Mrs. G. was a 90 year-old female living in a senior apartment building. She had rheumatoid arthritis, diabetes, dementia, and needed help with all activities of daily living. She had her son move into her apartment, allegedly to care for her; this was in violation of her lease which permitted only one tenant to reside in the apartment. Both the manager and several tenants reported that the son frequently brought different women to the apartment, and even sent Mrs. G. across the hall to a neighbor so he could have privacy. There were numerous complaints of guests coming and going at all hours, loud music and conversations late in the evening, and the smell of marijuana coming from the apartment–all of this in an apartment complex designed to insure the safety of seniors. The building manager finally served Mrs. G. with an eviction notice because the neighbors' rights were being violated.

A Final Caution: Assuring Mental Competence

One cannot overemphasize the importance of a thorough mental examination before deciding that an elder is indeed mentally competent. As families and home health care workers can attest, many elders can maintain a facade of mental competence for short periods of time. Mrs. F. was a 93 year-old female, living alone in the upper flat of her two-family income home. She was diabetic, had high blood pressure, rheumatoid arthritis, anemia, and was confined to a wheelchair. She could afford to hire a private caregiver but preferred to manage by herself. Mrs. F. had been examined previously by her physician and a protective services worker, both of whom said they found her to have no mental problems.

However, home care workers who saw her on a regular basis were aware that her mental competence was transitory. Her tenant who lived downstairs reported to the home care team that Mrs. F. did not follow a proper diet and often forgot to eat or take her medication. On one occasion, the tenant found Mrs. F. on the kitchen floor with the gas stove running most of the day. Mrs. F. remembered none of these incidences. Finally, protective services conducted a full psychosocial assessment, examining Mrs. F.'s physical well-being, emotional state of mind, and safety at home alone.

This time, the protective service worker visited on several occasions, at different times of the day, over an 8 week period; often there were pills spilled, a smell of urine, and Mrs. F. could not remember whether or not she had eaten or taken her medications. It was determined that Mrs. F. was unable to make appropriate decisions for herself; guardianship or placement in a 24-hour care facility were recommended. The tenant agreed to become Mrs. F.'s legal guardian and assume responsibility for her health care and personal needs. In such instances, a short interview is not sufficient to uncover underlying mental problems and a much more thorough mental evaluation may be required.

CONCLUSION

We have discussed examples of 3 types of self-neglect in the elderly: self-destructive behavior, non-compliance, and Diogenes Syndrome, primarily in instances in which the elder is mentally competent and capable of caring for him/herself. The view that elders have an unlimited right to choose their life style must be tempered by the impact which these actions have upon the communities with which these elders interact. We have described three types of communities: emotionally close communities, with which an individual interacts and with which s/he shares a common sense of identification or belonging; geographic communities, in which the individual resides; and emotionally detached communities, such as the service community, with which an individual interacts–perhaps frequently–but with which s/he shares little sense of identity or belonging.

We have suggested that different types of self-neglect are likely to impact each of these communities differently. The greatest impact is likely to occur with emotionally close communities, as an elder's family and close friends become distressed if s/he lives in filth or refuses to follow medical prescriptions. The geographic community will be most affected by Diogenes Syndrome, which may intrude upon the health and safety of neighbors. Self-neglect is likely to impact on an emotionally detached, or service community, only in those instances in which the neglectful elder's behavior impinges on the specific agency's area of operation, such as misuse of oxygen for the providing company, or failure to take medications for the physician. However, we have also noted that extreme cases of Diogenes Syndrome may take symptoms of their pattern with them even into clinics or hospitals.

With regard to solutions, we have suggested that there are ways of responding to community concerns without resorting to the common approach of declaring an elder to be demented and enforcing a change of environment. These include the enforcement of public health codes to cut down noxious weeds or spray for rats or roaches. At the extreme, service agencies may cut off services to clients who consistently refuse to observe required regimens. While agencies typically resist such actions, they may be necessary in some instances for the safety of the agency's own personnel and the community at large.

Finally, the pattern of extreme self-neglect raises several important issues which service providers must resolve in working with elderly self-neglect clients. Central to the situation is the degree to which individual rights and autonomy and responsibility to one's community conflict with each other. Does the individual actually have a responsibility to the community to carry out normal health and safety activities, such as keeping his/her home and person reasonably clean, not smoking in the presence of oxygen, and so on? Can an individual do whatever s/he wishes, even put life and limb in jeopardy, so long as s/he does not seek help from the community? How much autonomy can an individual be expected to relinquish in return for assistance? What is the impact of chronic self-neglect on the morale of the service community, as well as the family and other informal helpers? It is likely that extreme self-neglect threatens more than the neglectful individual him/herself, in that elderly clients who come after may receive less effective services from a demoralized service community.

REFERENCES

Baker, A A. (1976). Slow euthanasia–or "she will be better off in hospital." *British Medical Journal, 2*, 571-572.

Broom, L., Selznick, P., & Broom, D. (1984). *Essentials of sociology.* (3rd ed.). Itasca, IL: Peacock.

Burr, C. (1997). The AIDS exception: Privacy vs. public health. *The Atlantic Monthly, 279*, 57-67.

Clark, A. N., Mankikar, G. D., & Gray, I. (1975). Diogenes syndrome. A clinical study of gross neglect in old age. *Lancet, 1*, 366-368.

Cole, A. J., Gillett, T. P., & Fairbairn, A. (1992). A case of senile self-neglect in a married couple: "Diogenes a deux"? *International Journal of Geriatric Psychiatry, 7*, 839-841.

Duke, J. (1991). A national study of self-neglecting adult protective services clients. In T. Tatara & M. M. Rittman (Eds.), K.J. Kaufer Flores (Coordinator). *Findings of five elder abuse studies* (pp. 23-53). Washington, DC: National Aging Resource Center on Elder Abuse.

Henslin, J. M. (1999). *Sociology: A Down to Earth Approach.* Boston: Allyn and Bacon.

Howard, R. & Bergmann, K. (1993). Personality disorders in old age. *International Review of Psychiatry, 5*, 469-475.

Jackson, G. A. (1997). Diogenes syndrome–How should we manage it? *Journal of Mental Health, 6*, 113-116.

Kastenbaum, R., & Mishara, B. (1971). Premature death and self-injurious behavior in old age. *Geriatrics, 26*, 71-81.

Longres, J. F. (1994). Self-neglect and social control: A modest test of an issue. *Journal of Gerontological Social Work, 22*(3/4): 3-20.

Macmillan, D., & Shaw, P. (1966). Senile breakdown in standards of personal and environmental cleanliness. *British Medical Journal, 2,* 1032-1037.

Nelson, F., & Farberow, F. (1977). Indirect suicide in the elderly chronically ill. In K. A. Achte & J. Lonnquist (Eds). *Suicide research* (pp. 125-139). Helsinki: Psychiatria Fennica.

Orrell, M. W., Sahakian, B. J., & Bergmann, K. (1989). Self-neglect and frontal lobe dysfunction. *British Journal of Psychiatry, 155,* 101-105.

Pies, R. W., & Popli, A. P. (1995). Self-injurious behavior: Pathophysiology and implications for treatment. *Journal of Clinical Psychiatry, 56,* 580-588.

Radebaugh, T. S., Hooper, F. J., & Gruenberg, E. M. (1987). The social breakdown syndrome in the elderly population living in the community: The helping study. *British Journal of Psychiatry, 151,* 341-346.

Reed, P. G., & Leonard, V. E. (1989). An analysis of the concept of self-neglect. *Advances in Nursing Science, 12,* 39-53.

Roe, P. F. (1977). Self-neglect. *Age and Aging, 6,* 192-194

Sullivan, T. J., & Thompson, K. S. (1988). *Introduction to Social Problems.* New York: Macmillan.

Thomasma, D. C. (1984). Freedom and dependency in the very old. *Journal of the American Geriatrics Society, 32,* 906-914.

Ungvari, G. S., & Hantz, P. M. (1991a). Social breakdown in the elderly, I. Case studies and management. *Comprehensive Psychiatry, 32,* 440-444.

Ungvari, G. S., & Hantz, P. M. (1991b). Social breakdown in the elderly, II. Sociodemographic data and psychopathology. *Comprehensive Psychiatry, 32,* 445-449.

Wrigley, M., & Cooney, C. (1992). Diogenes syndrome–An Irish Series. *Irish Journal of Psychological Medicine, 9,* 37-41.

Index

Numbers followed by "f" indicate figures; "t" following page numbers indicate tables.

AA. *See* Alcoholics Anonymous
Abuse
  alcohol. *See* Alcohol abuse
  elder, 6
Adams, W. L., 58-59,65
Adult Protective Services (APS), 2,35
  and patient advocacy, 42-45
Advance Directives, 51
Age, as factor in self-neglect, 6-7
Aging
  as assault on dignity, 41-42
  and erosion of health, 40-41
  ethics and, confronting abuse and self-neglect in the elderly, 33-54. *See also* Self-neglect, in the elderly, ethical issues related to
Alcohol, physical dependence on, 60
Alcohol abuse
  behavior reinforcement due to, 60
  effect on thiamine absorption, 62
  in the elderly
    causes of, 59-60
    pharmacology of, 60
    prevalence of, 55,57-59
  and self-neglect, 7
  and self-neglect in the elderly, 55-75
  diagnosis of, 64-68,66t
  introduction to, 55-60
  Korsakoff's psychosis due to, 66
  neglect of basic needs, 61-62,61t, 63t
  neglect of psychosocial needs, 61t, 63-64
  neglect of safety needs, 61t, 62-63

  screening for, 64-68,66t
  treatment of, 68-71,70f
    AA in, 69
    brief interventions in, 68-69,70f
    detoxification in, 69,71
    follow-up from, 71
    structured interventions in, 69
    Wernicke-Korsakoff syndrome due to, 62
    Wernicke's encephalopathy due to, 62
  systemic effects on, 62,63t
  tolerance resulting from, 60
"Alcohol use disorders," defined, 57
Alcohol Use Disorders Identification Test (AUDIT), 65
Alcoholic Anonymous (AA), 69
Alcoholism
  definitions of, 56-57
  "milieu limited," 59
  types of, 59,64
Allen, S. A., 46-47
Alternative suicide, 23
Autonomy
  assessing decisional capacity and, 45-47
  personal, defined, 40-41
  and right to refuse treatment, 47-48
  vs. beneficience, 47-50

Baker, A., 8,14,15
Baker, F., 3,10
Barboriak, J. J., 58-59
Barry, K. L., 59
Basic needs, neglect of, among elderly

who abuse alcohol, 61-62, 61t,63t
Behavior(s)
indirect life-threatening, in the elderly, 79
indirect self-destructive, in the elderly, 79
life-threatening, indirect, in the elderly, 21-32. See also Elderly, indirect life-threatening behavior in; Indirect life-threatening behavior, in the elderly
self-injurious, in the elderly, 79
self-neglect–related, 2
and refusal of treatment, 48-50
suicidal, indirect, self-neglect as, 10-11
Behavior reinforcement, alcohol and, 60
Beneficence
competency, and paternalism, 50-52
defined, 50
vs. patient autonomy, 47-50
Bien, T. H., 68
Blondell, R. D., 55
Bok, S., 38
British Medical Journal
Buerger's disease, self-neglect in patients with, 24

Cabinet for Human Resources, 43
"CAGE questionnaire," 65
Capacity for self-care, 79
Capacity to decide, in self-neglect, 12
Caro, F. G., 24
Cassel, C., 40
Categorical Imperative, 40
Clark, A., 3,7,8-9,14,15
Clark, W. B., 57
Cloninger, C. R., 10,59
Cole, A., 5
Community(ies)
effects of self-neglect in the elderly on, 77-93. See also Self-neglect, in the elderly, community effects of
assuring mental competence prior to community involvement, 90
differential impact on, 84-88
enforcing public health codes, 88
eviction in, 89-90
handling community concerns, 88-90
importance of, 81
removal of services in, 89
emotionally close communities, effects of self-neglect in the elderly on, 83,85-86
emotionally close community, effects of self-neglect in the elderly on, 84-85
geographic, effects of self-neglect in the elderly on, 83,85-86
overlap of, effects of self-neglect in the elderly on, 87-88
service, effects of self-neglect in the elderly on, 83-84,86-87
types of, effects of self-neglect in the elderly on, 82-84
Competence, mental, assurance of, prior to community intervention, 90
Competency
beneficence, paternalism and, 50-52
defined, 50-51
Control, personal, in indirect self-destructive and life-threatening behavior, 25-26
Cooney, C., 6,14,15,16
Crooks, J., 25
Cruzan, N., 48
Cruzan v. Director, 48
Cyr, M. G., 65
Czirr, R., 10

Death of spouse, and self-neglect, 10
Deception, ethics of, 37-38
Decision-making capacity, assessment of, and autonomy, 45-47
Dementia, and self-neglect, 7
Depression, and self-neglect, 10
Devor, E. J., 59
Diabetes mellitus, self-neglect associated with, 23-24
"Diathesis-stress model of mental illness," 9-10
DiClemente, C. C., 67
Dignity
　aging as assault on, 41-42
　defined, 38-39
　in ethical treatment of the elderly, 36
　presentation of, 38-39
"Diogenes a deux," 80
Diogenes syndrome, 3,4
　enforcing public health codes related to, 88
　extreme form of, 80
Dyer, C., 14

Eccentricity, self-neglect and, 39-40
Elder abuse, 6
Elderly
　ethical treatment of
　　dignity in, 36
　　neglect in, 36
　　truth in, 36
　indirect life-threatening behavior in, 21-32
　　case report, 26-29
　　conceptualization of, 24-26
　　discussion, 29-31
　　indirect self-destructive and life-threatening behavior in, 25
　　introduction to, 22
　　literature review related to, 22-24
　　noncompliance in, 25
　lifestyles of, eccentricity and self-neglect, relationship between, 39-40
　self-abuse in, 5-7
　self-neglect in
　　alcohol abuse and, 55-75. *See also* Alcohol abuse, and self-neglect in the elderly
　　community effects of. *See also* Self-neglect, in the elderly, community effects of
　　community effects on, 77-93
　　ethical issues related to, 33-54. *See also* Self-neglect, in the elderly, ethical issues related to
　　senile breakdown in, 2,9
　　values of, eccentricity and self-neglect, relationship between, 39-40
Encephalopathy(ies), Wernicke's, alcohol abuse and, 62
Erskine, H., 2
Ethic(s)
　and aging, confronting abuse and self-neglect, 33-54
　of deception, 37-38
Ethical issues, in self-neglect, 12-13
　in the elderly, 33-54. *See also* Self-neglect, in the elderly, ethical issues related to
Eviction, self-neglect–related, 89-90
Ewing, J. A., 65

Fabian, 23
Fairburn, A., 5
Farberow, N., 11, 22-23
Fleming, M. F., 59
Friedmann, P. D., 71

Gallager, D., 10
Gender, as factor in self-neglect, 8
Gerber, K., 24
Gillet, T., 5
Graham, K., 58
Granick, R., 2

Gruenberg, E., 7
Gruman, C. A., 24

Hantz, P., 9
Health, aging effects on, 40-41
Henderson-Smith, S., 13,14
Henney, D., 25
Herranz, R., 40-41
"Hidden suicide," 23
Hoarding, self-neglect and, 10
Hyman, D., 44

Indirect life-threatening behavior, in the elderly, 21-32,79
  case report, 26-29
  conceptualization of, 24-26
  discussion, 29-31
  indirect self-destructive and life-threatening behavior in, 25
  introduction to, 22
  literature review related to, 22-24
  noncompliance in, 25
Indirect self-destructive behavior (ISDB), in the elderly, 79
Intelligence, self-neglect and, 7
International Classification of Diseases, 9th Revision, in defining alcohol abuse and dependency, 56
Isolation, social, and self-neglect, 7

Jenkins, M., 29
Jonsen, A., 34

Kant, I., 40
Kastenbaum, R., 3
Kitchens, J. M., 65
Korsakoff's psychosis, alcohol abuse and, 66
Kuzmeskus, L., 6

Lachs, M., 15
Laird-Fick, H. S., 1
Legal issues, in self-neglect, 12-13
Leonard, V. E., 3,11,24,79
Life-Threatening behavior, indirect, in the elderly, 21-32. *See also* Elderly, indirect life-threatening behavior in; Indirect life-threatening behavior, in the elderly indirect, in the elderly, 21-32
Longres, F., 4,14,16
Longress, J., 24

MacMillan, D., 3,5,6,8,9,10,11,14,15, 16,23
Mental competence, assurance of, prior to community intervention, 90
Mental illness, "diathesis-stress model of," 9-10
Michigan Alcohol Screening Test (MAST), 65
Midanik, L. T., 57
Miller, C., 3,10
Miller, W. R., 68
Mishara, B., 3

National Association of Adult Protective Services Administrators (NAAPSA), 4
National Elder Abuse Incidence Study, 3
National Health Survey on Drug Abuse, 58
National Highway Traffic Safety Administration (NHTSA), in alcohol abuse, 63
National Institutes of Health, in defining alcohol abuse, 57
National Longitudinal Alcohol Epidemiologic Survey, 58
Nelson, F., 22-23
Neuropsychiatric disorders, and self-neglect, 10

Noncompliance, in indirect self-destructive and life-threatening behavior, 25
Norcross, J. C., 67
Northern, M. C., 45,46,50-51

O'Brien, J. G., 1, 21,33
Obsessive-compulsive disorder, self-neglect and, 10
Orem's self-care model, in self-neglect, 13

Parkin, D., 25
Passive suicide, in indirect self-destructive and life-threatening behavior, 25
Paternalism
  beneficence, and competency, 51-52
  defined, 51
Patient advocacy, Adult Protective Services in, 42-45
Patient as person, in ethical treatment of the elderly, 38-39
Personal control, in indirect self-destructive and life-threatening behavior, 25-26
Physical dependence, alcohol and, 60
Pies, R., 10
Planned Parenthood of SE Pennsylvania v. Case, 48
"Police Rubber Bullets End," 45
Popli, A., 10
Post, F., 9
Prochaska, J. O., 67
Psychosis, Korsakoff's, alcohol abuse and, 66
Psychosocial needs, neglect of, among elderly who abuse alcohol, 61t, 63-64
Public health codes, community enforcement of, 88

Quirk, J., 25

Race, age as factor in, 6-7
Radebaugh, T., 3
Rathbone-McCuan, D., 32
Rathbone-McCuan, R. E., 29
Reed, P. G., 3,11,24,79
Refusal of treatment, self-neglecting behavior and, 48-50
Respect for the person, in ethical treatment of the elderly, 36
Right to refuse treatment, autonomy and, 47-48
Rimm, A. A., 58-59
Roe, P., 14,15

Safety needs, neglect of, among elderly who abuse alcohol, 61t, 62-63
Saitz, R., 71
Samet, J. H., 71
Schillinger, B., 44
Self-abuse. *See also* Self-neglect
  in the elderly, 5-7
  social isolation and, 7
Self-care, capacity for, 79
Self-injurious behavior (SIB), in the elderly, 79
Self-neglect. *See also* Self-abuse
  age as factor in, 6-7
  alcohol abuse and, 7
  background of, 2-5
  behaviors associated with, 2,48-50. *See also under* Behavior(s)
  in Buerger's disease, 24
  causes of, 8-11
  comorbidities associated with, 7
  concept of, 1,2
  death of spouse and, 10
  defined, 4,56-57
  definitional problems associated with, 2
  dementia and, 7
  described, 4
  detection of, 11

in diabetics, 23-24
and eccentricity, 39-40
in the elderly
  alcohol abuse and, 55-75. *See also*
      Alcohol abuse, and
      self-neglect in the elderly
    case example, 34-36
    community effects of, 77-93.
        See also Community(ies),
        effects of self-neglect in the
        elderly on differential impact
        on, 84-88
      introduction to, 77-79
    ethical issues related to, 33-54
      Adult Protection Services in,
          42-45
      assault on dignity, 41-42
      autonomy, 45-47
      beneficence, 50-52
        vs. autonomy, 47-48
      competency, 50-52
      decision-making capacity of
          patient, 45-47
      dignity in, 36,38-39
      ethics of deception, 37-38
      introduction to, 33-34
      paternalism, 51-52
      patient advocacy, 42-45
      respect for the person, 36
      treatment, 37-38
      truth in, 36,38-39
    indirect life-threatening behavior,
        21-32. *See also* Elderly,
        indirect life-threatening
        behavior in; Indirect
        life-threatening behavior, in
        the elderly
      types of, 79-80
  epidemiology of, 5-8
  ethical issues related to, 12-13
  in the elderly, 33-54. *See also*
      Self-neglect, in the elderly,
      ethical issues related to
  extreme form of. *See* Diogenes
      syndrome
  gender as factor in, 8
  hoarding in, 10
  incidence of, 5-6
  as indirect suicidal behavior,
      10-11
  intelligence and, 7
  interventions in, 13-15
  legal issues related to, 12-13
  living alone and, 7
  management of, 13-15
  neuropsychiatric disorders and,
      10
  obsessive-compulsive disorder
      and, 10
  Orem's self-care model in, 13
  outcome of, 15-16
  overview of, 1-19
  pre-morbid characteristics of,
      8-9
  prevention of, 16-17
  profile of victim of, 8
  race as factor in, 6-7
  social isolation and, 7
Self-neglecting behavior. *See under*
    Behavior(s)
Selzer, M. L., 65
Sengstock, M. C., 77
Senile breakdown in the elderly
    (SBE), 2
  overall picture of, 9
Senile breakdown syndrome, 3,5
Shaw, P., 2,5,6,8,9,10,11,14,15,16,23
Short Michigan Alcohol Screening
    Test (SMAST), 65
Siegler, M., 34
Simmons, P. D., 33
Social breakdown in the elderly, 80
Social breakdown syndrome, 4
Social isolation, and self-neglect, 7
Spouse, death of, and self-neglect, 10
State of Tennessee Department of
    Human Services v. Mary C.
    Northern, 45
Stern, A. S., 24
Subintentional suicide, 23
Substance Abuse and Mental Health
    Services Adminstration
    (SAMHSA), 58

Suicidal behavior, indirect,
    self-neglect as, 10-11
Suicidal equivalent, 23
Suicide
    alternative, 23
    hidden, 23
    passive, in indirect self-destructive
        and life-threatening behavior,
        25
    subintentional, 23
        alternative, 23
Supreme Court of Tennessee, 45

Tarasoff v. Regents of the University
    of California, 51
Tatara, T., 6
The Physicians' Guide to Helping
    Patients with Alcohol
    Problems, 70f
"The Roby Ridge Standoff," 45
Thiamine absorption, alcohol
    inhibition and, 62
Thibault, J. M., 1,10,21,26,77
Thompson, L., 10
Tolerance, alcohol and, 60
Tonigan, J. S., 68
Truth
    in ethical treatment of the elderly,
        36
    and patient as person, in ethical
        treatment of the elderly,
        38-39
Turner, L. C., 1, 21

Ungvari, G., 9
Union Pacific Railway Company v.
    Botsford, 48

Van Rooijen, L., 65
Vinokur, A., 65

Wartment, S.A., 65
Wernicke-Korsakoff syndrome,
    alcohol abuse and, 62
    treatment of, 69-70
Wernicke's encephalopathy, alcohol
    abuse and, 62
Whitehead, T., 9
Winslade, W., 34
World Health Organization, in
    defining alcohol abuse and
    dependency, 57
Wrigley, M., 6,14,15,16

Yuan, Z., 58-59

Zaranek, R., 77
Zeman, F., 2